ABC OF DERMATOLOGY

ABC OF DERMATOLOGY

SECOND EDITION

PAUL K BUXTON FRCPED, FRCPC

Consultant dermatologist
Royal Infirmary, Edinburgh, and Fife Health Board

with contributions from

D J GAWKRODGER, D W S HARRIS,
D KEMMETT, A L WRIGHT

Published by the BMJ Publishing Group
Tavistock Square, London WC1H 9JR

First published 1988
Second impression 1989
Third impression 1990
Fourth impression 1991
Fifth impression 1991
Second edition 1993
Second impression 1994
Third impression 1994

British Library Cataloguing in Publication Data

Buxton, P K
    ABC of dermatology.
  1. Medicine. Dermatology
    British Medical Journal: 0007-1447
    616.5

ISBN 0-7279-0758-1

Printed in Singapore, by Craft Print Pte Ltd
Typesetting by Apek Typesetters, Avon House, Blackfriars Road, Nailsea, Bristol BS19 2DJ

Contents

INTRODUCTION

The object of this book is to provide the non-specialist with a practical guide to the diagnosis and treatment of skin conditions. The symptoms, clinical appearance, and pathology of a few key common conditions are discussed. These are then used as a model for comparison with other skin diseases.

This approach is suitable for skin conditions that present with characteristic lesions such as blisters, ulceration, papules, or a rash. In other disorders, where there may be a single causative factor that produces a variety of lesions, it is more helpful to describe the characteristic clinical pattern that results; allergic reactions, autoimmunity, and infection are examples. Tumours, acne, and leg ulcers are covered as separate subjects.

One advantage of dealing with skin conditions is that the lesions are easily examined and can be interpreted without the need for complex investigations, although biopsy is sometimes required to make or confirm the diagnosis. An understanding of the histological changes underlying the clinical presentation makes this interpretation easier and more interesting. Consequently, clinical descriptions are accompanied by an account of the underlying pathological changes.

Skin lesions are sometimes an indication of internal disease and may be the first clinical sign. For example, the girl in the photograph presented with a rash on her face, made worse by sunlight. She then mentioned that she was aware of lassitude, weight loss, and vague musculoskeletal symptoms which, in conjunction with the appearance of the rash, suggested lupus erythematosus. This was confirmed by further investigations and appropriate treatment initiated. Other dermatological associations with systemic disease are discussed in the relevant sections.

Lupus erythematosus.

Descriptive terms

All specialties have their own common terms, and familiarity with a few of those used in dermatology is a great help. The most important are defined below.

Macule

Derived from the Latin for a stain, the term macule is used to describe changes in colour or consistency without any elevation above the surface of the surrounding skin. There may be an increase of melanin, giving a black or blue colour depending on the depth of the pigment. Loss of melanin leads to a white macule. Vascular dilatation and inflammation produce erythema.

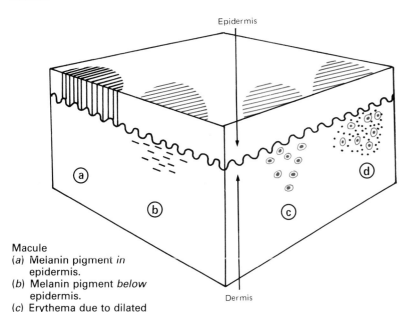

Epidermis

Dermis

Macule
(a) Melanin pigment *in* epidermis.
(b) Melanin pigment *below* epidermis.
(c) Erythema due to dilated dermal blood vessels.
(d) Inflammation in dermis.

Introduction

Papules and nodules

5mm

15mm

A papule is a circumscribed, raised lesion, conventionally less than 1 cm in diameter. It may be due to either epidermal or dermal changes.

A nodule is similar to a papule but over 1 cm in diameter.

Plaque

Plaque is one of those terms which convey a clear meaning to dermatologists but are often not understood by others. To take it literally, one can think of a commemorative plaque stuck on the wall of a building with a large area relative to its height and a well defined edge. Plaques are most commonly seen in psoriasis.

Vesicles and bullae

Vesicles and bullae are raised lesions that contain fluid. A bulla is a vesicle larger than 0·5 cm. They may be superficial within the epidermis or situated in the dermis below it.

Lichenification

Lichenification is another term frequently used in dermatology as a relic of the days of purely descriptive medicine. Some resemblance to lichen seen on rocks and trees does occur, with hard thickening of the skin and accentuated skin markings. It is most often seen as a result of prolonged rubbing of the skin in localised areas of eczema.

Nummular lesions

The word nummular literally means a "coin like" lesion. There is no hard and fast distinction from *discoid* lesions, which are flat disc like lesions of variable size. It is most often used to describe a type of eczematous lesion.

Pustules

The term pustule is applied to lesions containing purulent material—which may be due to infection, as in the case shown, or sterile pustules are seen in pustular psoriasis.

Atrophy

Loss of tissue may affect the epidermis, dermis, or subcutaneous fat. Thinning of the epidermis is characterised by loss of the normal skin markings, and there may be fine wrinkles, loss of pigment, and a translucent appearance. There may be other changes as well, such as sclerosis of the underlying connective tissue, telangectasia, or evidence of diminished blood supply.

Ulcer

Ulceration results from the loss of the whole thickness of the epidermis and upper dermis. Healing results in a scar.

Erosion

An erosion is a superficial loss of epidermis that generally heals without scarring.

Excoriation

Excoriation is the partial or complete loss of epidermis as a result of scratching.

Fissuring

Fissures are slits through the whole thickness of the skin.

Introduction

Annular lesions

Annular lesions are ring shaped lesions.

Reticulate

The term reticulate means "net like." It is most commonly seen when the pattern of subcutaneous blood vessels become visible

Rashes

Psoriasis of both legs.

(Above) Symmetrical rash—irritant dermatitis.

(Left) Asymmetrical rash—contact dermatitis in a seamstress.

Allergic reactions producing photosensitivity. Note the areas protected by a vest in the patient on the right.

Approach to diagnosis

A skin rash generally poses more problems in diagnosis than a single, well defined skin lesion such as a wart or tumour. As in all branches of medicine a reasonable diagnosis is more likely to be reached by thinking firstly in terms of broad diagnostic categories rather than specific conditions.

If there is no history of a skin condition the rash is more likely to be due to an exogenous cause (such as contact dermatitis) than a constitutional condition (such as atopic eczema). Psoriasis can, however, appear in adults with no previous episodes. If several members of the household are affected a contagious condition should be considered (such as scabies). However, a common condition with a familial tendency, such as atopic dermatitis, may affect several family members at different times.

A simplistic but helpful approach to rashes is to clarify them as being from "inside" or "outside." Examples of "inside" or endogenous rashes are atopic eczema or drug rashes, whereas fungal infection or contact dermatitis are "outside" rashes. Although this distinction is not always clear cut, each type has distinctive characteristics.

Symmetry

Most endogenous rashes affect both sides of the body, as in the atopic child or man with psoriasis on his knees. Of course, not all exogenous rashes are asymmetrical. A seamstress uses scissors in her right hand, where she may develop allergy to metal, but a hairdresser or nurse can develop contact dermatitis on both hands.

Distribution

It is useful to be aware of the usual sites of common skin conditions. These are shown in the appropriate sections. Eruptions that appear only on areas exposed to sun may, of course, be entirely or partially due to sunlight. Some conditions are due to a sensitivity to sunlight alone, such as polymorphous light eruption, or a photosensitivity to topically applied substances or drugs taken internally.

4

Lesion in deeper tissues with normal epidermis.

Small vesicles of eczema.

Morphology

The appearance of the skin lesion may give clues to the underlying pathological process.

The surface may consist of normal epidermis overlying a lesion in the deeper tissues. This is characteristic of many types of erythema in which there is dilatation of the dermal blood vessels associated with inflammation. The skin overlying cysts or tumours in the dermis and deeper tissues is usually normal. Conditions affecting the epidermis will produce several visible changes such as thickening of the keratin layer and scales in psoriasis or a more uniform thickening of the epidermis in areas lichenified by rubbing. An ezcematous process is characterised by small vesicles in the epidermis with crusting or fine scaling.

The margin of some lesions is very well defined, as in psoriasis or lichen planus, but in eczema it merges into normal skin.

Eczema—intraepidermal vesicle

Intraepidermal vesicle with residual nuclei

"Spongiosus"—oedema between epidermal cells

Blisters or vesicles occur as a result of (*a*) oedema between the epidermal cells or (*b*) destruction of epidermal cells or (*c*) the result of separation of the epidermis from the deeper tissues. Of course, more than one mechanism may occur in the same lesion. Oedema within the epidermis is seen in endogenous eczema, although it may not be apparent clinically, particularly if it is overshadowed by inflammmation and scaling. It is also a feature of contact dermatitis. Widespread blisters occur in:

(*a*) viral diseases such as chickenpox; hand, foot, and mouth disease; and herpes simplex;

(*b*) bacterial infections such as impetigo;

(*c*) primary blistering disorders such as dermatitis herpetiformis, pemphigus, pemphigoid, metabolic disorders such as porphyria.

Pemphigus—destruction of epidermal cells

Acantholysis—separation and destruction of the epidermal cells

Bullae may occur in congenital conditions (such as epidermolysis bullosa), lichen planus, and pemphigoid without much inflammation. On the other hand, those forming as a result of vasculitis, sunburn, or an allergic reaction may be associated with pronounced inflammation. In pustular psoriasis there are deeper pustules, which contain polymorphs but are sterile and show little inflammation. Drug rashes can appear as a bullous eruption.

Induration is thickening of the skin due to infiltration of cells; granuloma formation; or deposits of mucin, fat, or amyloid.

Inflammation is indicated by erythema, which may be accompanied by increased temperature if acute—for example, in cellulitis or erythema nodosum. Chronic inflammatory cells may be present in conditions such as lichen planus or lupus eythematosus.

Pemphigoid—blister forming below epidermis

Subepidermal blister

Inflammatory infiltrate

Pemphigus—superficial blister.

Herpes simplex.

Impetigo.

Dermatitis herpetiformis.

Introduction

Assessment of the patient

A relevant history should be taken with particular reference to:

Where? Site of initial lesion(s) and subsequent distribution.

How long? Has the condition been continuous or intermittent?

Prognosis Is it getting better or worse?

Previous episodes How long ago? Were they similar? Have there been other skin conditions?

Who else? Are other members of the family affected? Or colleagues at work or school?

Other features Is there itching, burning, scaling, or blisters? Any associated factors, drugs, associated illnesses? Any effect of occupation, or home environment?

Treatment By prescription or over the counter?

Patients should be examined with particular reference to:

Distribution—This may give the essential clue, so a full examination is necessary. For example, there are many possible causes for dry thickened skin on the palms, and finding typical psoriasis on the elbows, knees, and soles may give the diagnosis.

Morphology—Are the lesions dermal or epidermal? Macular (flat) or forming papules? Indurated or forming plaques? With a well defined edge? Forming crusts, scabs, or vesicles?

Pattern—This is the overall clinical picture of both morphology and distribution. For example, an indeterminate rash may be revealed as pityriasis rosea when the "herald patch" is found.

We now come to the matter of using these basic concepts in the diagnosis of lesions in practice. In the next four chapters two common skin diseases are considered—psoriasis, which affects 1–2% of the population, and eczema, an even more common complaint. Both are rashes with epidermal changes. The difficulty arises with the unusual lesion: Is it a rarity or a variation of a common disease? What should make us consider further investigation? Is it safe to wait and see if it resolves or persists? The usual clinical presentations of psoriasis and eczema are also used as a basis for comparison with variations of the usual pattern and other skin conditions.

The effect of a skin condition of the patient's life and the patient's attitude to it must always be taken into account. For example, severe pustular psoriasis of the hands can be devastating for a self employed electrician and total hair loss from the scalp very distressing for a 16 year old girl.

Fear that a skin condition may be due to cancer or infection is often present and reassurance should always be given whether asked for or not. If there is the possibility of a serious underlying cause that requires further investigation it is part of good management to answer any questions the patient has and provide an explanation that he or she can understand. We all forget this aspect of medical practice at times.

The role of occupational factors must be remembered: dermatitis of the hands often means a hairdresser must change her job whereas it may be readily controlled in a teacher.

Patients understandably ask whether psoriasis can be cured and often want to know the cause. The cause is unknown and the best answer is that the tendency to develop psoriasis is part of a person's constitution and some factor triggers the development of the clinical lesions. Known factors include physical or emotional stress, local trauma to the skin (Koebner's phenomenon), infection (in guttate psoriasis), drugs (β blockers, lithium, and antimalarial drugs).

6

PSORIASIS

Increased epidermal proliferation—nuclei found . . . throughout the epidermis

The familiar pink or red lesions with a scaling surface and well defined edge are easily recognised. These changes can be related to the histological appearance.

(1) The increased thickness of the epidermis, presence of nuclei above the basal layer, and thick keratin are related to increased epidermal turnover.

(2) Because the epidermis is dividing it does not differentiate adequately into normal keratin scales. These are readily removed to reveal the tortuous blood vessels beneath—clinically, "Auspitz sign." The psoriatic plaque can be likened to a brick wall badly built by a workman in too much of a hurry—it may be high but it is easily knocked down.

(3) The polymorphs that migrate into the epidermis form sterile pustules in pustular psoriasis. These are most commonly seen on the palms and soles.

(4) The dilated blood vessels can be a main feature, giving the clinical picture of intense erythema.

The equivalent changes in the nail cause thickening and "pits" 0·5–1·0 mm in diameter on the surface; these are thought to be due to small areas of psoriatic changes in the upper nail plate that then fall out.

While still considering the individual lesion remember the following points.

Plaques of psoriasis.

The *size* of the lesions varies from a few millimetres to very extensive plaques.

Scaling may predominate, giving a thick plaque, which is sometimes likened to limpets on the sea shore, hence the name "rupioid." Scratching the surface produces a waxy appearance—the "tache de bougie" (literally "a line of candle wax").

Erythema may be conspicuous, especially in lesions on the trunk and flexures.

Pustules are rare on the trunk and limbs, but deep seated pustules on the palms and soles are fairly common.

Pitting of nail.

Small and large lesions.

Rupioid lesions

Widespread pustular psoriasis.

Pustules on the sole.

Psoriasis

The typical patient

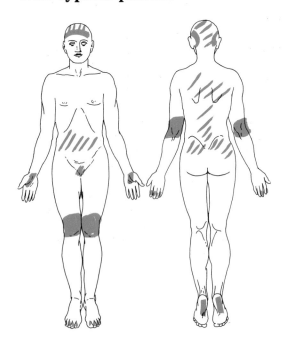

Psoriasis usually occurs in early adult life, but the onset can be at any time from infancy to old age, when the appearance is often atypical. The following factors in the history may help in making a diagnosis.

- There may be a family history—if one parent has psoriasis 25% of the children will have it, if both parents the figure is 60%.
- The onset can occur after any type of stress, including infection, trauma, or childbirth
- The lesions may first appear at sites of minor trauma—Koebner's phenomenon
- The lesions usually clear on exposure to the sun
- Typically, psoriasis does not itch
- There may be associated arthropathy—affecting either the fingers and toes or a single large joint.

Clinical presentation

Patients usually present with plaques and sometimes annular lesions on the elbows, knees, and scalp. Patients with psoriasis show Koebner's phenomenon with lesions developing in areas of skin trauma such as scars or minor scratches. Normal everyday trauma such as handling heavy machinery may produce hyperkeratotic lesions on the palms. In the scalp there is scaling, sometimes producing very thick accretions. Erythema often extends beyond the hair margin. The nails show "pits" and also thickening with separation of the nail from the nail bed (oncholysis).

Annular lesons.

Koebner's phenomenon: psoriasis in surgical scar.

Psoriasis of the nail.

Variations

Guttate psoriasis.

Flexural psoriasis.

Pustules on the foot.

Napkin psoriasis.

Guttate psoriasis—from the Latin *gutta*, a drop—consists of widespread small pink macules that look like drops of paint. It usually occurs in adolescents and often follows an acute β haemolytic streptococcal infection. There may be much distress to both parent and child when a previously healthy adolescent erupts in apparent leprous spots.

Pustular lesions occur as chronic deep seated lesions on the palms and soles with surrounding erythema which develop a brown colour and scaling. In clinics north of the border these pustules make the patient ask whether the condition is "smitten"—that is, infectious. It is important always to explain that it is not.

Flexural psoriasis produces well defined erythematous areas in the axillae and groins and beneath the breasts. Scaling is minimal or absent.

Napkin psoriasis in children may present with typical psoriatic lesions or a more diffuse erythematous eruption with exudative rather than scaling lesions.

8

Scalp psoriasis.

Erythrodermic psoriasis.

Generalised pustular psoriasis is uncommon. Superficial pustules develop in an area of intense erythema.

Erythrodermic psoriasis is a serious, even life threatening, condition with erythema affecting nearly the whole of the skin. Diagnosis may not be easy as the characteristic scaling of psoriasis is absent, although this usually precedes the erythroderma. Less commonly the erythema develops suddenly without preceding lesions. There is a considerable increase in cutaneous blood flow, heat loss, metabolism, and water loss.

It is important to distinguish between the stable, chronic, plaque type of psoriasis, which is unlikely to develop exacerbations and responds to tar, dithranol, and ultraviolet treatment, and the more acute erythematous type, which is unstable and likely to spread rapidly, particularly when irritated by tar, dithranol, or ultraviolet light.

Joint disease in psoriasis

Acute arthropathy.

Patients with seronegative arthropathy of the non-rheumatoid type show double the normal (2%) incidence of psoriasis. Psoriatic arthropathy commonly affects the distal interphalangeal joints, sparing the metacarpophalangeal joints, and is usually asymmetrical. Rheumatoid nodules are absent. The sex ratio is equal but a few patients develop a "rhematoid like" arthropathy, which is more common in women than in men. There is a third rare group who suffer from arthritic changes, in which there is considerable resorption of bone.

Other members of the families of those with psoriatic arthropathy are affected in 40% of cases.

There may be severe pustular psoriasis of the fingers and toes associated with arthropathy. One patient was so severely affected that she was immobilised until her condition cleared on treatment with methotrexate.

Cause of psoriasis

There is evidence that both hormonal and immunological mechanisms are involved at a cellular level. The raised concentrations of metabolites of arichodonic acid in the affected skin of people with psoriasis are related to the clinical changes. Prostaglandins cause erythema, while leukotrienes (LTB4 and 12 HETE) cause neutrophils to accumulate. The common precursor of these factors is phospholipase A2, which is influenced by calmodulin, a cellular receptor protein for calcium. Both phospholipase A2 and calmodulin concentrations are raised in psoriatic lesions.

T helper lymphocytes have been found in the dermis as well as antibodies to the basal cell nuclei of psoriatic skin. There are also dermal factors that contribute to the development of psoriatic lesions.

> **Hormonal and immunological mechanisms and dermal factors are involved in the development of psoriasis**

The detailed treatment of psoriasis is covered in the next chapter. The only point to be made here is the importance of encouraging a positive attitude with expectation of improvement but not a permanent cure, since psoriasis can recur at any time. Some patients are unconcerned about very extensive lesions while to others the most minor lesions are a catastrophe.

TREATMENT OF PSORIASIS

Presentation of psoriasis	Treatment of choice	Alternative treatment
Stable plaque	Short contact dithranol	Tar
Extensive stable plaque	PUVA+etretinate	Short contact dithranol
Widespread small plaque	Ultraviolet B	Tar
Guttate psoriasis	Emollients while erupting then ultraviolet B	Weak tar preparations
Facial psoriasis	1% Hydrocortisone ointment	
Flexural psoriasis	Local mild to moderate strength steroids+ antifungal	
Pustular psoriasis of hands and feet	Moderate to potent strength local steroid	Etretinate
Acute erythrodermic, unstable, or generalised pustular psoriasis	Inpatient treatment with ichthammol paste. Local steroids may be used in skilled hands	Methotrexate

To ignore the impact of the condition on the patient's life is to fail in treating psoriasis. Like the Cheshire cat that Alice met, it tends to clear slowly and the last remaining patches are often the hardest to clear.

This is frustrating enough but there is also the knowledge that it will probably recur and need further tedious courses of treatment. So encouragement and support are an essential part of treatment.

Treatment comprises local treatment with ointments and pastes, systemic drugs, or various forms of ultraviolet light. Treatment should suit the type of psoriasis. The age and health of the patient and social and occupational factors need to be taken into consideration. The motivation of the individual patient is also important.

The preparations mentioned in the text are listed in the formulary at the end of the book.

Local treatment

Local treatments entail the use of ointments and pastes, usually containing tar in various forms. It is much easier to apply them in hospital than at home if patients can make the time for hospital visits. Inpatient treatment can be more intensive and closely regulated; it also has the advantage of taking the patient completely away from the stresses of the everyday environment. In some units a "five day ward" enables patients to return home at weekends, which is particularly important for parents with young children.

Coal tar preparations are safe and effective for the stable plaque-type psoriasis but will irritate acute, inflamed areas. On the other hand, tar may not be strong enough for thicker hyperkeratotic lesions. Salicylic acid, which helps dissolve keratin, can be used in conjunction with tar for thick plaques. Refined coal tar extracts can be used for less severe areas of psoriasis.

Ichthammol, prepared from shale rather than coal tar, is less irritating and has a soothing effect on inflamed skin. It is therefore useful for "unstable" or inflamed psoriasis, when tar would not be tolerated.

Short contact dithranol

Indications—Stable plaque psoriasis on the trunk and limbs.

Suitable preparations—Those available in a range of concentratons such as Dithocream (0·1%, 0·25%, 0·5%, 1·0%, 2·0%) or Anthranol (0·4%, 1·0%, 2·0%).

Method—(1) Start with the lowest concentration and increase strength every 5 to 6 days if there are no problems. (2) Apply cream to affected areas and then wash it off completely 20 to 30 minutes later. (3) Apply a bland emollient immediately after treatment.

Cautions—(1) Do *not* apply to inflamed plaques, flexures, or the face. (2) Avoid contact of the dithranol with clothing and rinse the bath well after use to avoid staining. (3) Never leave the cream on for longer than 30 minutes. (60 minutes is not twice as effective.)

Dithranol, obtained originally from the Goa tree in south India, is now made synthetically. It can easily irritate or burn the skin, so it has to be used carefully and should be kept from contact with normal skin as far as possible. For hospital treatment pastes are used and the lesions surrounded by vaseline to protect the normal skin. Dithranol creams can be used at home—they are applied for 30 minutes and then washed off. A low concentration (0.1%) is used initially and gradually increased to 1% or 2% as necessary. All dithranol preparations are irritants and produce a purple-brown staining that clears in time. If used in the scalp it stains red or fair hair purple.

Emollients soften dry skin and relieve itching. They are a useful adjunct to tar or dithranol.

Corticosteroid preparations produce an initial clearing of psoriasis, but there is rapid relapse when they are withdrawn and tachyphylaxis (increasing amounts of the drug have a diminishing effect) occurs. Strong topical steroids should be avoided. Only weak preparations should be used on the face but moderately potent steroids can be used elsewhere if there are only a few small lesions of psoriasis; if there is persistent chronic psoriasis of the palms, soles, and scalp (in conjunction with tar paste, which is applied on top of the steroid at night); and in the treatment of psoriasis of the ears, flexures, and genital areas. In flexural psoriasis secondary infection can occur and steroid preparations combined with antibiotics and antifungal drugs should be used, such as Terra-Cortril with nystatin and Trimovate.

Calcipotriol is a vitamin D analogue used as an ointment for mild or moderate plaque psoriasis.

Psoriasis suitable for short contact dithranol treatment.

Ultraviolet treatment

Guttate psoriasis suitable for ultraviolet B treatment.

Ultraviolet B is short wavelength ultraviolet light and is used for widespread thin lesions or guttate psoriasis. The dose has to be accurately controlled to give enough radiation to clear the skin without burning.

Ultraviolet A is long wavelength ultraviolet light, which is effective if combined with systemic psoralens (PUVA): 8-methoxypsoralen (0·6–0·8 mg/kg body weight) is taken one to two hours before treatment.

After medical assessment treatment is given two or three times a week, with gradually increasing doses of ultraviolet A, given in a specially designed cabinet. Once the psoriasis has been cleared maintenance treatments can be continued once every two or three weeks. Protective goggles are worn during treatment with ultraviolet A and opaque glasses for 24 hours after each treatment.

PUVA cabinet.

Treatment of psoriasis

Before PUVA.　　　After PUVA.

A variable degree of erythema and itching may occur after treatment. Longer term side effects include a slight risk of epitheliomas developing, premature aging of the skin, and cataract formation (which can be prevented by wearing ultraviolet A filtering goggles during and after treatment). The total cumulative dosage is carefully monitored and kept as low as possible to reduce the risk of side effects.

Systemic treatment

Erythematous psoriasis suitable for methotrexate treatment, having failed to respond to PUVA.

Extensive and inflamed psoriasis that is resistant to local treatment may require systemic treatment. Although a number of antimetabolite drugs (such as azathioprine and hydroxyurea) and immunosuppressive drugs (such as cyclosporin A) are used, methotrexate and etretinate are the most useful.

Methotrexate inhibits folic acid synthesis during the S phase of mytosis and diminishes epidermal turnover in the lesions of psoriasis. Because it is hepatotoxic liver function has to be assessed initially and at regular intervals during treatment. The dosage must be monitored and when a total of 1·5 g is reached a liver biopsy is indicated to exclude significant liver damage. An initial test dose is followed by a test for full blood count and if this gives normal results a weekly dose of 7·5–15 mg is used. As it is excreted in the urine the dose must be reduced if renal function is impaired. Aspirin and sulphonamides diminish plasma binding. It may interact with barbiturates, para-aminobenzoic acid, phenytoin, probenecid, phenylbutazone, oral contraceptives, and colchicine.

Etretinate is a vitamin A derivative that can be prescribed only in hospital in the United Kingdom. It is useful in pustuar psoriasis but has limited effect on other types of psoriasis. However, the effect is increased when combined with PUVA. Minor side effects include drying of the mucous membranes, crusting in the nose, itching, thinning of the hair, and erythema of the palms and nail folds. These are usually not severe and settle when treatment stops. More significant side effects include hepatotoxicity and raised lipid concentrations. Liver function tests and serum lipid (cholesterol and triglyceride) concentrations have to be carefully monitored. Etretinate is teratogenic and should not normally be used in women during reproductive years. If it is used effective contraception must be used during treatment and for two years afterwards as the half life is 70–100 days.

Psoriasis of the scalp

- Scalp psoriasis can be very difficult to clear, particularly if there are thick scales

- 3% Salicylic acid is a suitable base and can be left on for four to six hours or overnight and then washed out with a tar shampoo

- Dithranol preparations are effective but tint blonde or red hair purple

- Steroid preparations can be used to control itching.

ECZEMA AND DERMATITIS

Eczema.

The terms eczema and dermatitis are interchangeable, covering a wide variety of conditions from the child with atopic eczema to the adult with an allergy to cement. "Eczema" is more specific and in some countries indicates a more acute condition than "dermatitis." If patients are told they have dermatitis they may assume that it is related to their employment with the implication that they may be eligible for compensation. It is not unusual for industrial workers to ask "Is it dermatitis doctor?"—meaning "is it due to my job?"

Clinical appearance

Eczema is an inflammatory condition of the skin characterised by groups of vesicular lesions with a variable degree of exudate and scaling. In some cases dryness and scaling predominate with little inflammation. In more acute cases there may be considerable inflammation and vesicle formation, in keeping with the Greek for "to boil out," from which the word eczema is derived. Sometimes the main feature may be blisters that can become very large.

Eczema commonly itches and the clinical appearance may be modified by scratching, which with time may produce lichenification (thickening of the skin with increased skin markings). Also as a result of scratching the skin surface may be broken and have excoriations, exudate, and secondary infection.

Eczema—intraepidermal vesicle

Intraepidermal vesicle with residual nuclei

"Spongiosus"—oedema between epidermal cells

Pathology

The characteristic change is oedema between the cells of the epidermis, known as spongiosus, leading to formation of vesicles. The whole epidermis becomes thickened with an increased keratin layer. A variable degree of vasodilatation in the dermis and an inflammatory infiltrate may be present.

Types of eczema

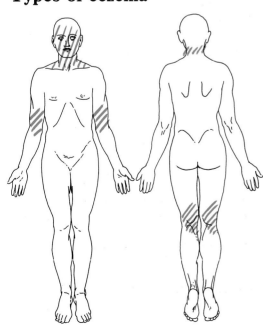
Atopic eczema.

The many causes of eczema are not consistently related to the distribution and clinical appearance. In general there are either external factors acting on the skin producing inflammatory changes or it is an endogenous condition. It is important to remember there can be more than one cause—for example, in atopic eczema or varicose eczema on the ankle an additional allergic reaction may develop to the treatments used.

Atopic eczema.

Nummular eczema.

Eczema and dermatitis

Plantar dermatosis.

Atopic eczema affects mainly the flexor surfaces of the elbows and knees and the face and neck. To a variable degree it can afect the trunk as well.

The typical patient with atopic eczema is a fretful scratching child with eczema that varies in severity, often from one hour to the next. In the older child or adult eczema is more chronic and widespread and its occurrence is often related to stress. Atopic eczema is common, affecting 3% of all infants, and runs a chronic course with variable remissions. It normally clears during childhood but may continue into adolescence and adult life as a chronic disease. It is often associated with asthma and rhinitis. Sufferers from atopic eczema often have a family history of the condition.

Variants of atopic eczema are pityriasis alba—white patches on the face of children with a fair complexion—and chronic juvenile plantar dermatosis—dry cracked skin of the forefoot in children. This does not affect the interdigital spaces and is not due to a fungal infection.

Eczema herpeticum—Children with atopic eczema are particularly prone to herpes virus infection, which may be life threatening. Close contact with adults with "cold sores" should therefore be avoided.

Nummular eczema appears as coin shaped lesions on legs and trunk.

Stasis eczema occurs around the ankles, where there is impaired venous return.

Paget's disease of the breast—While eczema of the nipples and areolae occur in women, any *unilateral*, persistent, areas of dermatitis in this region may be due to Paget's disease, in which there is underlying carcinoma of the ducts. In such cases a biopsy is essential.

Nummular eczema.

Stasis eczema.

Paget's disease of the nipple.

Lichen simplex.

Lichen simplex is a localised area of lichenificaton produced by rubbing.

Neurodermatitis is a term often used synonymously with lichen simplex. It is also used to describe generalised dryness and itching of the skin, usually in those with atopic eczema.

Asteatotic eczema occurs in older people with a dry, "crazypaving" pattern, particularly on the legs.

Pompholyx is itching vesicles on the fingers, with lesions on the palms and soles in some patients.

Infection can modify the presentation of any type of eczema or contact dermatitis.

Asteatosis.

Pompholyx.

Infected eczema.

Contact dermatitis

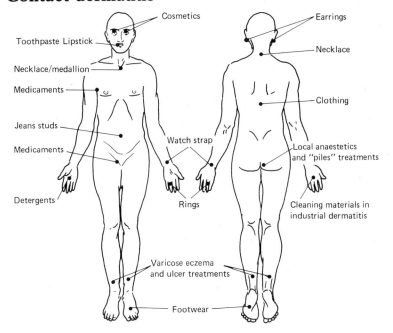

Common sources of allergic contact dermatitis

Jewellery, clothing, wristwatch, scissors, cooking utensils	Nickel—and cobalt occasionally
Cement, leather	Chromate
Hair dyes, tights, shoes	Paraphenylenediamine
Rubber gloves and boots	Rubber preservative chemicals
Creams, ointments, cosmetics	Preservatives (para-benzquarternium), balsam of Peru, fragrances, lanolin neomycin, benzocaine, in medicated ointments

Allergic reactions to: (top left) topical neomycin; (right) dithranol; (bottom left) Solarcaine and sun; and (right) sulphapyridine by mouth.

Irritant reaction to bleach.

The skin normally performs its function as a barrier very effectively. If this is overcome by substances penetrating the epidermis an inflammatory response may occur leading to epidermal damage. These changes may be due to either (a) an allergic response to a specific substance acting as a sensitiser or (b) a simple irritant effect. An understanding of the difference between these reactions is helpful in the clinical assessment of contact dermatitis.

The characteristics of allergic dermatitis are (a) previous exposure to the substance concerned; (b) 48 to 96 hours between contact and the development of changes in the skin; (c) activation of previously sensitised sites by contact with the same allergen elsewhere on the body; and (d) persistence of the allergy for many years.

Allergic contact dermatitis can be illustrated by the example of an individual with an allergy to nickel who has previously reacted to a wrist watch. Working with metal objects that contain nickel leads to dermatitis on the hands and also a flare up at the site of previous contact with the watch. The skin clears on holiday but the dermatitis recurs two days after the person returns to work.

On the other hand, *irritant contact dermatitis* has a much less defined clinical course and is caused by a wide variety of substances with no predictable time interval between contact and the appearance of the rash. Dermatitis occurs soon after exposure and the severity varies with the quantity, concentration, and length of exposure to the substance concerned. Previous contact is not required, unlike allergic dermatitis where previous sensitisation is necessary.

Photodermatitis, caused by the interaction of light and chemical absorbed by the skin, occurs in areas exposed to light. It may be due to (a) drugs taken internally, such as sulphonamides, phenothiazines, and dimethylchlortetracycline, or (b) substances in contact with the skin, such as topical antihistamines, local anaesthetics, cosmetics, and antibacterials.

Morphology—The clinical appearance of both allergic and irritant contact dermatitis may be similar but there are specific changes that help in differentiating them. An acute allergic reaction tends to produce erythema, oedema, and vesicles. The more chronic lesions are often lichenified. Irritant dermatitis may present as slight scaling and itching or extensive epidermal damage resembling a superficial burn, as the child in the illustration shows.

Pathology—The allergic reaction to specific sensitisers leads to a typical eczematous reaction with oedema separating the epidermal cells and blister formation. In irritant dermatitis there may also be eczematous changes but also non-specific inflammation, thickening of keratin, and pyknotic, dead epidermal cells.

Eczema and dermatitis

Allergic reactions to: (left) rubber pad on goggles; (middle) cosmetics; and (above) elastic in underpants.

Photodermatitis.   Leg dermatitis.

The distribution of the skin changes is often helpful. For example, an itchy rash on the waist may be due to an allergy to rubber in the waistband of underclothing or a metal fastener. Gloves or the rubber lining of goggles can cause a persisting dermatitis. An irritant substance often produces a more diffuse eruption, as shown by the patient who developed itching and redness from dithranol.

Photodermatitis can occur from everyday household substances such as soap—the man in the photograph reacted to the trichlorsalicalanilide in soap he had used before working in his garden. The outline of the area protected by his vest can be seen.

An allergy to medications used for treating leg ulcers is a common cause of persisting dermatitis on the leg. Common allergens are listed in the box.

Patch testing

Patch testing is used to determine the substances causing contact dermatitis. The concentration used is critical. If it is too low there may be no reaction, giving a false negative result, and if it is too high it may produce an irritant reaction, which is interpreted as showing an allergy (false positive). Another possible danger is the induction of an allergy by the test substance. The optimum concentration and best vehicle have been found for most common allergens, which are the basis of the "battery" of tests used in most dermatology units.

The test patches are left in place for 48 hours then removed, the sites marked, and any positive reactions noted. A further examination is carried out at 96 hours to detect any further reactions.

It is most important not to put a possible causative substance on the skin in a random manner without proper dilution and without control patches. The results will be meaningless and irritant reactions, which are unpleasant for the patient, may occur.

Classification of eczema

Endogenous (constitutional) eczema	*Exogenous (contact) eczema*	*Secondary changes*
• Atopic	• Irritant	• Lichen simplex
• Nummular/Discoid	• Allergic	• Neurodermatitis
• Pompholyx	• Photodermatitis	• Asteatosis
• Stasis		• Pompholyx
• Seborrhoeic (discussed later)		• Infection

TREATMENT OF ECZEMA AND INFLAMMATORY DERMATOSES

(1) Treat the patient, not just the rash

(2) Avoid promising complete cure

(3) Be realistic about applying treatments at home

(4) Make sure the patient understands how to carry out the treatment

(5) Advise using emollients and minimal soap

(6) Provide detailed guidance on using steroids

Weeping eczema.

Acute erythema.

Treat the patient, not just the rash. Many patients accept their skin condition with equanimity but others suffer much distress—especially if the face and hands are affected. Acceptance by the doctor of the individual and his or her attitudes to the disease goes a long way to helping the patient live with the condition.

The common inflammatory skin diseases can nearly always be improved or cleared—but it is wise not to promise a permanent cure.

Be realistic about the treatment people can apply in their own homes. It is easy to unthinkingly give patients with a widespread rash a large amount of ointment to apply twice daily, which is hardly used because: (a) they have a busy job or young children and simply do not have time to apply ointment to the whole skin; (b) they have arthritic or other limitations of movement and can reach only a small part of the body; (c) the tar or other ointment is smelly or discolours their clothes. Most of us have been guilty of forgetting these factors at one time or another.

Dry skin tends to be itchy, so advise minimal use of soap. Emollients are used to soften the skin, and the simpler the better. Emulsifying ointment *BP* is cheap and effective but rather thick. I advise patients to mix two tablespoons in a kitchen blender with a pint of water—the result is a creamy mixture that can easily be used in the bath. A useful preparation is equal parts of white soft paraffin and liquid paraffin. Various proprietary bath oils are available and can be applied directly to wet skin. This is more sensible than putting them in the bath water, which makes the bath slippery with more oil going down the drain than on the skin. There are many proprietary emollients.

Steroid ointments are effective in relieving inflammation and itching but are not always used effectively. Advise patients to use a strong steroid (such as betamethasone or fluocinolone acetonide) frequently for a few days to bring the condition under control; then change to a weaker steroid (dilute betamethasone, fluocinolone, clobetasone, hydrocortisone) less frequently. Strong steroids should not be continued for long periods, and do not prescribe any steroid stronger than hydrocortisone for the face as a rule. Strong steroids can cause atrophy of the skin if used for long periods, particularly when applied under occlusive dressings. On the face they may lead to florid telangiectasia and acne like pustules. Avoid using steroids on ulcerated areas. Prolonged use of topical steroids may mask an underlying bacterial or fungal infection.

Specific treatment

Wet, inflamed, exuding lesions

(1) Use wet soaks with normal saline or aluminium acetate (0·6%). Potassium permanganate (0·1%) solution should be used if there is any sign of infection.

(2) Use wet compresses rather than dry dressings.

(3) Steroid *creams* should be used as outlined above. Greasy ointment bases tend to float off on the exudate.

(4) A combined steroid-antibiotic cream is often needed as infection readily develops.

(5) Systemic antibiotics may be required in severe cases. Take swabs for bacteriological examination first.

Treatment of eczema and inflammatory dermatoses

Lichenified eczema.

Dry, scaling, lichenified lesions

(1) Use emollients.

(2) Use steroid *ointments*, with antibiotics if infection is present.

(3) A weak coal tar preparation or ichthammol can be used on top of the ointments. This is particularly useful at night to prevent itching. 1–2% Coal tar can be prescribed in an ointment. For hard, lichenified skin salicylic acid can be incorporated and the following fomulation has been found useful in our department: coal tar solution *BP* 10%, salicylic acid 2%, and unguentum drench to 100%. 1% Ichthammol and 15% zinc oxide in white soft paraffin is less likely to irritate than tar and is suitable for children.

(4) In treating psoriasis start with a weaker tar preparation and progress to a stronger one.

(5) For thick, hyperkeratotic lesions, particulary in the scalp, salicylic acid is useful. It can be prescribed as 2–5% in aqueous cream, 1–2% in arachis oil, or 6% gel.

It is often easiest for the patient to apply the preparation to the scalp at night and wash it out the next morning with a tar shampoo.

Infection

Remember that secondary infection may be a cause of persisting lesions.

Hand dermatitis

Infected eczema. Before and after treatment.

Hand dermatitis: hints on management

(1) Hand washing:
Use tepid water and soap without perfume or colouring or chemicals added. Dry carefully, especially between fingers.

(2) When in wet work:
Wear cotton gloves under rubber gloves (or plastic if you are allergic to rubber). Try not to use hot water and cut down to 15 minutes at a time if possible. Remove rings before wet or dry work. Use running water if possible.

(3) Wear gloves in cold weather and for dusty work.

(4) Use only ointments prescribed for you.

(5) Things to avoid:
(a) Shampoo
(b) Peeling fruits and vegetables, especially citrus fruits
(c) Polishes of all kinds
(d) Solvents—eg, white spirit, thinners, turpentine
(e) Hair lotions, creams, and dyes
(f) Detergents and strong cleansing agents
(g) "Unknown" chemicals.

(6) Use "moisturisers" or emollients which have been recommended by your doctor—to counteract dryness.

Hand dermatitis poses a particular problem in management and it is important that protection is continued after the initial rash has healed since it takes some time for the skin to recover its barrier function. Ointments or creams should be reapplied each time the hands have been washed.

It is useful to give patients a list of simple instructions such as those shown here.

Management of pruritus (itching skin)

Causes

Endocrine diseases—Diabetes, myxoedema, hyperthyroidism.

Metabolic diseases—Hepatic failure, chronic renal failure.

Malignancy—Lymphoma, reticulosis, carcinomatosis.

Psychological—Anxiety, parasitophobia.

Tropical Infection—Filariasis, hookworm.

Drugs—Alkaloids.

Scratching the skin produces lichenification so that it is not always possible to know if there was originally an underlying area of eczema or another primary itching condition of the skin.

Endogenous eczema can produce severe itching, often made worse by secondary infection. Irritants or allergens also cause an intense itching and should be suspected, particularly if the eyelids or hands are affected.

Scabies causes intense itching and can be overlooked. Take scrapings for mycological examination. In the absence of any other apparent condition remember the causes of pruritus shown in the box.

Treatment—The object of symptomatic treatment is to break the "itch-scratch-itch" cycle once the cause has been eliminated. Topical steroid ointments and occulusive dressings help to prevent scratching.

Use emollients for dry skin.

Topical local anaesthetics give relief but can cause allergic reactions. Sedative antihistamines at night may be helpful.

In liver failure cholestyramine powders may help to relieve the intense pruritus that can occur.

Pruritus ani is a common, troublesome condition and the following points may be helpful.

(1) Patients often wash obsessively and attack the perianal area frequently with soap and water. Advise gentle cleaning, once daily.

(2) Avoid harsh toilet paper—especially if it is coloured (cheap dyes irritate and can cause allergies). Olive oil and cotton wool can be used instead.

(3) Weaker topical steroids can be used to reduce inflammation with zinc cream or ointment as a protective layer on top.

(4) Anal leakage from an incompetent sphincter, skin tags, or haemorrhoids may require surgical treatment.

(5) There may be anxiety or depression but pruritus ani itself can lead to irritability and depression.

RASHES WITH EPIDERMAL CHANGES

Lichen planus
Seborrhoeic dermatitis
Pityriasis rosea
Pityriasis lichenoides
Localised lesions

Familiarity with the clinical features of psoriasis and eczema, which all clinicians see from time to time, provides a basis for comparison with other rather less common conditions.

The characteristics that each condition has in common with psoriasis and eczema are highlighted.

Lichen planus

Clinical features of psoriasis	Clinical features of eczema
Possible family history	Possible family history
Sometimes related to stress	Sometimes worse with stress
Itching—rare	Usually itching
Extensor surfaces and trunk	Flexor surfaces and face
Well defined, raised lesions	Poorly demarcated lesions
Hyperkeratosis	Oedema, vesicles, lichenificaton
Scaling, bleeding points beneath scales	Secondary infection sometimes present
Koebner's phenomenon	
Nails affected	
Scalp affected	
Mucous membranes not affected	

Like psoriasis, the lesions are well defined and raised. They also occur in areas of trauma—Koebner's phenomenon. There is no constant relation to stress. *Unlike* psoriasis, there is no family history. Itching is common. The distribution is on the flexor aspects of the limbs, particularly the ankles and wrists, rather than on the extensor surfaces, as in psoriasis. However, localised forms of lichen planus can occur on the shin, palm, and soles or elsewhere.

The typical flat topped lesions have a shiny hyperkeratotic lichenified surface with a violaceous colour, interrupted by milky white streaks—Wickham's striae. The oral mucosa is commonly affected with a white, net like appearance and sometimes ulceration.

Lichen planus—oral mucosa.

Lichen planus—nail.

Lichhen planus—skin.

Lichen planus.

Less commonly very thick hypertrophic lesions occur and also follicular lesions. Lichen planus is one cause of localised alopecia on the scalp as a result of hair follicle destruction.

Nail disease is less common than in psoriasis. There may be thinning and atrophy of part or all of a nail and these often take the form of a longitudinal groove.

Lichen planus usually resolves over many months to leave residual brown or grey macules. In the oral mucosa and areas subject to trauma ulceration can occur.

Lichenified eczema.

Guttate psoriasis.

Similar rashes

Lichenified eczema—This is also itchy and may occur on the ankles and wrists. The edge of the lesion is less well defined and is irregular. The flat topped, shiny papules are absent.

Guttate psoriasis is not as itchy as lichen planus. Scaling erythematous lesions do not have the lichenified surface of lichen planus.

Pityriasis lichenoides—The lesions have a mica like scale overlying an erythematous papule.

Drug eruptions—Rashes with many features of lichen planus can occur in patients taking:

Chloroquine ⎫
Chlorpropamide ⎬ The 3 "C"s
Chlorothiazide ⎭
Anti-inflammatory drugs
Gold preparations

It also occurs in those handling colour developers.

Treatment

The main symptom of itching is relieved to some extent by moderately potent steroid ointments. Very hypertrophic lesions may respond to strong steroid preparations under polythene occlusion. Careful intralesional injections may be very effective in persistent lesions. In very extensive, severe lichen planus systemic steroids may be indicated.

Lichen planus

Flexor surfaces
Mucous membranes affected
Itching common
Violaceous colour
Wickham's striae
Small discrete lesions
Lichenified

Lichenified eczema.

Guttate psoriasis.

— Hyperkeratosis
— Increase in granular layer
— Cellular infiltrate
— Degeneraton of basal layer

Pathology of lichen planus

As expected from the clinical appearance, there is hypertrophy and thickening of the epidermis with increased keratin. The white streaks seen clinically occur where there is pronounced thickness of the granular layer and underlying infiltrate. Degenerating basal cells may form "colloid bodies." The basal layer is being eaten away by an aggressive band of lymphocytes, the remaining papillae having a "saw toothed" appearance.

Seborrhoeic dermatitis

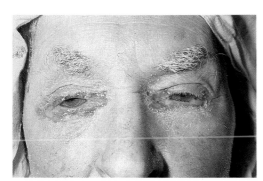

Seborrhoeic dermatitis.

Seborrhoeic dermatitis has nothing to do with sebum or any other kind of greasiness. There are two distinct types, adult and infantile.

Adult seborrhoeic dermatitis

The adult type is more common in men and in those with a tendency to scaling and dandruff in the scalp. There are several commonly affected areas.

(*a*) Seborrhoeic dermatitis affects the central part of the face, scalp, ears, and eyebrows. There may be an associated blepharitis, giving some red eyes and also otitis externa.

(*b*) The lesions over the sternum sometimes start as a single "medallion" lesion. A flower like "petaloid" pattern can occur. The back may be affected as well.

(*c*) Lesions also occur in well defined areas in the axillae and groin and beneath the breasts.

Rashes with epidermal changes

Seborrhoeic dermatitis.

Typically the lesions are discrete and erythematous and they may develop a yellow crust. The lesions tend to develop from the hair follicles. It is a persistent condition that varies in severity.

Clinically and pathologically the condition has features of both psoriasis and eczema. There is thickening of the epidermis with some of the inflammatory changes of psoriasis and the intercellular oedema of eczema. Parakeratosis—the presence of nuclei above the basement layer—may be noticeable. In recent years an increased number of *Pityrasporum ovale*, a normal commensal yeast, have been found.

Treatment—Topical steroids produce a rapid improvement, but not permanent clearing. Topical preparations containing salicylic acid, sulphur, or ichthammol may help in long term control. Triazole antifungal drugs by mouth have been reported to produce clearing and can be used topically. These drugs clear yeasts and fungi from the skin, including *P ovale*, which is further evidence for the role of this organism.

Clinical featues of psoriasis	Clinical features of eczema
Possible family history	Possible family history
Sometimes related to stress	Sometimes worse with stress
Itching—rare	Usually itching
Extensor surfaces and trunk	Flexor surfaces and face
Well defined, raised lesions	Poorly demarcated lesions
Hyperkeratosis	Oedema, vesicles, lichenification
Scaling, bleeding points beneath scales	Secondary infection sometimes present
Koebner's phenomenon	
Nails affected	
Scalp affected	
Mucous membranes not affected	

Infantile seborrhoeic dermatitis

In infants less than 6 months old a florid red eruption occurs with well defined lesions on the trunk and confluent areas in the flexures associated with scaling of the scalp. There is no consistent association with the adult type of seborrhoeic dermatitis. It has been suggested that infantile seborrhoeic dermatitis is a variant of atopic eczema. A high proportion of affected infants develop atopic eczema later but there are distinct differences. It is said to be more common in bottle fed infants.

Treatment comprises applying emollients, avoiding soap, and applying hydrocortisone combined with an antibiotic plus nystatin (for example, Terra-Cortril plus nystatin cream). Hydrocortisone can be used on the scalp.

Infantile seborrhoeic dermatitis.

Itching is present in atopic eczema but not in seborrhoeic dermatitis.

The clinical course of atopic eczema is prolonged with frequent exacerbations, whereas seborrhoeic dermatitis clears in a few weeks and seldom recurs.

Allergy—IgE concentrations are often raised in atopic eczema and food allergy is common, but not in seborrhoeic dermatitis.

Perioral dermatitis

Perioral dermatitis is possibly a variant of seborrhoeic dermatitis, with some features of acne. Papules and pustules develop around the mouth and chin. It occurs mainly in women.

Perioral dermatitis.

Pityriasis rosea

Lichen planus
Seborrhoeic dermatitis

Pityriasis rosea
Pityriasis lichenoides
Localised lesions

Herald lesions.

Clinical featues of psoriasis	Clinical features of eczema
Possible family history	Possible family history
Sometimes related to stress	Sometimes worse with stress
Itching—rare	Usually itching
Extensor surfaces and trunk	Flexor surfaces and face
Well defined, raised lesions	Poorly demarcated lesions
Hyperkeratosis	Oedema, vesicles, lichenification
Scaling, bleeding points beneath scales	Secondary infection sometimes present
Koebner's phenomenon	
Nails affected	
Scalp affected	
Mucous membranes not affected	

The word "pityriasis" is from the Greek for bran, and the fine bran like scales on the surface are a characteristic feature. The numerous pale pink oval or round patches can be confused with psoriasis or discoid eczema. The history helps since this condition develops as an acute eruption and the patient can often point to a simple initial lesion—the herald patch.

There is commonly slight itching. Pityriasis rosea occurs mainly in the second and third decade, often during the winter months. "Clusters" of cases occur but not true epidemics. This suggests an infective basis. There may be prodromal symptoms with malaise, fever, or lymphadenopathy. Numerous causes have been suggested from allergy to fungi; the current favourite is a virus infection.

The typical patient is an adolescent or young adult, who is often more than a little concerned about the sudden appearance of a widespread rash. The lesions are widely distributed, often following skin creases, and concentrated on the trunk with scattered lesions on the limbs. The face and scalp may be affected.

Early lesions are red with fine scales— usually 1–4 cm in diameter. The initial herald patch is larger and may be confused with a fungal infection. Subsequently the widespread eruption develops in a matter of days or, rarely, weeks. As time goes by the lesions clear to give a slight pigmentation with a collarette of scales facing towards the centre.

Similar rashes

Discoid eczema presents with itching and lesions with erythema, oedema, and crusting rather than scaling. Vesicles may be present. The rash persists unchanged.

A *drug eruption* can sometimes produce similar lesions.

Guttate psoriasis—The lesions are more sharply defined and smaller (0·5–1·0 cm) and have waxy scales.

The pathology of pityriasis rosea

Histological changes are non-specific, showing slight inflammatory changes in the dermis, oedema, and slight hyperkeratosis.

Pityriasis lichenoides

Pityriasis lichenoides is a less common condition occurring in acute and chronic forms.

The *acute* form presents with widespread pink papules which itch and form crusts, sometimes with vesicle formation suggestive of chickenpox. There may be ulceration. The lesions may develop in crops and resolve over a matter of weeks.

The *chronic* form presents as reddish brown papules—often with a "mica" like scale that reveals a smooth, red surface underneath, unlike the bleeding points of psoriasis. In lichen planus there is no superficial scale and blistering is unusual.

The distribution is over the trunk, thighs, and arms, usually sparing the face and scalp.

Rashes with epidermal changes

A mica scale pityriasis lichenoides.

The underlying pathology—vascular dilatation and a lymphocytic infiltrate with a keratotic scale—is in keeping with the clinical appearance. The cause is unknown. Treatment is with topical steroids.

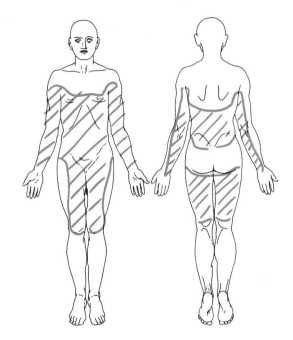

Clinical featues of psoriasis	Clinical features of eczema
Possible family history	Possible family history
Sometimes related to stress	Sometimes worse with stress
Itching—rare	Usually itching
Extensor surfaces and trunk	Flexor surfaces and face
Well defined, raised lesions	Poorly demarcated lesions
Hyperkeratosis	Oedema, vesicles, lichenification
Scaling, bleeding points beneath scales	Secondary infection sometimes present
Koebner's phenomenon	
Nails affected	
Scalp affected	
Mucous membranes not affected	

Pityriasis versicolor

Pityriasis versicolor is a skin eruption that usually develops after sun exposure with white macules on the tanned skin but pale brown patches on the covered areas—hence the name—versicolor, or variable colour. The lesions are: (*a*) flat; (*b*) only *partially* depigmented—areas of vitiligo are totally white; and (*c*) do not show inflammation or vesicles.

The causitive organism is a yeast—*Pityrosporum orbiculare*—that takes advantage of some unknown change in the epidermis and develops a proliferative, stubby, mycelial form—*Malassezia furfur*. This otherwise incidental information can be simply put to practical use by taking a superficial scraping from a lesion on to a microscope slide—add a drop of potassium hydroxide or water with a coverslip. The organisms are readily seen under the microscope: spherical yeast forms and mycelial rods, resembling "grapes and bananas" ("spaghetti and meatballs" in the United States).

Treatment is simple: selenium sulphide shampoo applied regularly with ample water while showering or bathing will clear the infection. The colour change may take some time to clear. Ketoconazole shampoo is an effective alternative. Oral terbinafine, which is very effective in other fungal infections, has no effect.

Desquamating stage of generalised erythema

Any extensive acute erythema, from the erythroderma of psoriasis to a penicillin rash, commonly shows a stage of shedding large flakes of skin—desquamation—as it resolves. If only this stage is seen it can be confused with psoriasis.

Localised lesions with epidermal changes

Flexural seborrhoeic dermatitis.

Psoriasis, seborrhoeic dermatitis, atopic eczema, and contact dermatitis can all present with localised lesions.

Psoriasis may affect only the flexures, occur as genital lesion, or affect only the palms. The lack of itching and epidermal changes with a sharp edge help in differentiation from infective or infiltrative lesions.

Corynebacterium minutissimum (erythrasma).

Seborrhoeic dermatitis can occur in the axillae or scalp with no lesions of other areas.

Atopic eczema—The "classical" sites in children—flexures of the elbows and knees and the face—may be modified to localised vesicular lesions on the hands and feet in older patients. Some atopic adults develop severe, persistent generalised eczematous changes.

Contact dermatitis is usually localised, by definition, to the areas in contact with irritant or allergen. Wide areas can be affected in reactions to clothing or washing powder, and sometimes the reaction extends beyond the site of contact.

Systemic lupus erythematosus.

Fungal infections—Apart from athlete's foot, toenail infections, and tinea cruris (in men) "ringworm" is in fact not nearly as common as is supposed. The damp, soggy, itching skin of athlete's foot is well known. An itching, red diffuse rash in the groin differentiates tinea cruris from psoriasis. However, erythrasma, a bacterial infection, may be confused with seborrhoeic dermatitis and psoriasis—skin scrapings can be taken for culture of *Corynebacterium minutissimum* or, more simply, coral pink fluorescence shown with Wood's light. The scaling macules from dog and cat ringworm (*Microsporum canis*) itch greatly while the indurated pustular, boggy lesion (kerion) of cattle ringworm is quite distinctive.

Fungal infection of the axillae is rare; a red rash here is more likely to be due to erythrasma or seborrhoeic dermatitis.

Tinea cruris is very unusual before puberty and is uncommon in women.

In all cases of suspected fungal infection skin scrapings should be taken on to black paper, in which they can be folded and sent to the laboratory. In some units special "kits" are provided, which contain folded black paper and Sellotape strips on slides for taking a superficial layer of epidermis.

Discoid lupus erythematosus.

Lupus erythematosus—There are two forms of this condition: *discoid*, which is generally limited to the skin, and *systemic*, in which the skin changes are associated with disease of the kidneys and other organs. The acute, erythematous rash on the malar area of the face, usually in a woman, is characteristic of the systemic type. In discoid lupus erythematosus there are well defined lesions, which are a combination of atrophy and hyperkeratosis of the follicles, giving a "nutmeg grater" feel. It occurs predominantly on the face or areas exposed to the sun as chronic, erythematous lesions that are much worse in the summer months.

Rashes with epidermal changes

Fixed drug eruption.

Fixed drug eruptions—Generalised drug eruptions are considered under erythema, but there is a localised form recurring every time the drug is used. There is usually a well defined, erythematous plaque, sometimes with vesicles. Crusting, scaling, and pigmentation occur as the lesion heals. It is usually found on the limbs, and more than one lesion can occur.

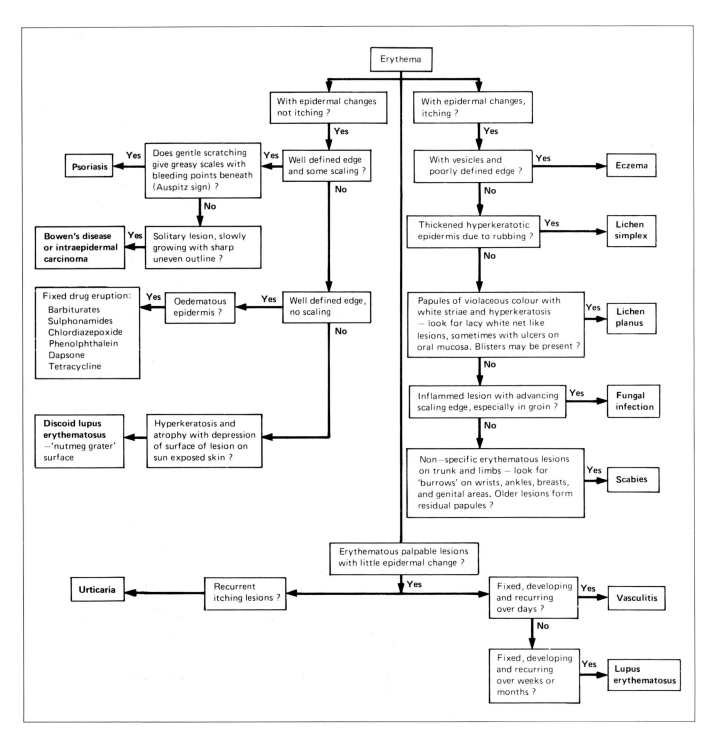

RASHES ARISING IN THE DERMIS

The erythemas

Erythema from antibiotics.

Complex reactions occuring in the capillaries and arterioles of the skin cause erythema— which is simply redness of the skin. This may present as flat macules or as papules, which are raised above the surrounding skin. The lesions may be transient or last for weeks, constant or variable in distribution, with or without vesicles.

It is possible to recognise specific patterns within this plethora of clinical signs, but even the most experienced dermatologist may be reduced to making a general diagnosis of "toxic" erythema. The best we can do therefore is to recognise the common types of erythema and list the possible causes. It is then a matter of deciding on the most likely underlying condition or group of conditions—for example, bacterial infection or autoimmune systemic disease.

Morphology and distribution

Because there can be the same cause for a variety of erythematous rashes detailed descriptions are of limited use. None the less, there are some characteristic patterns.

Morbilliform—The presentation of measles is well known, with the appearance of Koplik's spots on the mucosa, photophobia with conjunctivitis, and red macules behind the ears, spreading to the face, trunk, and limbs. The prodromal sysmptoms and conjunctivitis are absent in drug eruptions. Other viral conditions, including those caused by echoviruses, rubella, infectious mononucleosis, and erythema infectiosum may have to be considered.

Scarlatiniform rashes are similar to that in scarlet fever, when an acute erythematous eruption occurs in relation to a streptococcal infection. Characteristically erythema is widespread on the trunk. There is intense erythema and engorgement of the pharyngeal lymphoid tissue with an exudate and a "strawberry" tongue. Bacterial infections can produce a similar rash, as can drug rashes, without the systemic symptoms.

Figurate erythemas are chronic erythematous rashes forming annular or serpiginous patterns. There may be underlying malignancy or connective tissue disease.

Causes of "toxic" erythema

Drugs	antibiotics, barbiturates, thiazides
Infections	any recent infections such as streptococcal throat infection or erysipelas; spirochaetal infections; viral infections
Systemic causes	pregnancy; connective tissue disease; malignancy

---

Erythema multiforme

Erythema multiforme is sometimes misdiagnosed because of the variety of lesions and number of possible precipitating causes; some of these are listed below.

Erythema multiforme.

Infections	*Neoplasia*
Herpes simplex—the commonest cause	Hodgkin's disease
Mycoplasma infection	Myeloma
Infectious mononucleosis	Carcinoma
Poliomyelitis (vaccine)	*Chronic inflammation*
Many other viral and bacterial infections	Sarcoidosis
Any focal sepsis	Wegener's granuloma
BCG inoculaton	*Drugs*
Collagen disease	Barbiturates
Systemic lupus erythematosus	Sulphonamides
Polyarteritis nodosa	Penicillin
	Phenothiazine and many others

Rashes arising in the dermis

Annular lesions of erythema multiforme.

Clinical picture

The usual erythematous lesions occur in crops on the limbs and trunk. Each lesion may extend, leaving a cyanotic centre, which produces an "iris" or "target" lesion. Bullae may develop in the lesions and on the mucous membranes. A severe bullous form, with lesions on the mucous membranes, is known as the Stevens-Johnson syndrome. There may be neural and bronchial changes as well. Barbiturates, sulphonamides, and other drugs are the most common cause.

Histologically there are inflammatory changes, vasodilatation, and degeneration of the epidermis.

A condition that may be confused is *Sweet's syndrome*, which presents as acute plum coloured raised painful lesions on the limbs—sometimes the face and neck—with fever. It is more common in women. The alternative name, "acute febrile neutrophilic dermatosis," describes the presentation and the pathological findings of a florid neutrophilic infiltrate. There is often a preceding upper respiratory infection. Treatment with steroids produces a rapid response but recurrences are common.

Annular lesions of erythema multiforme.

Blistering lesions.

Erythema induratum

Erythema induratum occurs on the lower legs posteriorly, usually in women, with diffuse, indurated dusky red lesions that may ulcerate. It is more common in patients with poor cutaneous circulation. Epithelioid cell granulomas may form.

It was originally described in association with tuberculous infection elsewhere in the body (Bazin's disease). It represents a vasculitic reaction to the infection, and when there is no tuberculous infection another chronic infection may be responsible.

Erythema nodosum

Erythema nodosum occurs as firm, gradually developing lesions, predominantly on the extensor aspect of the legs. They are tender and progress from an acute erythematous stage to residual lesions resembling bruises over four to eight weeks.

Single or multiple lesions occur varying in size from 1 to 5 cm. The lesions are often preceded by an upper respiratory tract infection and may be associated with fever and arthralgia. Infections (streptococcal, tuberculous, viral, and fungal) and sarcoidosis are the commonest underlying conditions. Drugs can precipitate erythema nodosum, the contraceptive pill and the sulphonamides being the commonest cause. Ulcerative colitis, Crohn's disease, and lymphoma may also be associated with the condition.

Rashes due to drugs

Fixed drug eruption.

There is an almost infinite variety of types of drug reaction.

External contact with drugs can cause a contact dermatitis presenting with eczematous changes. This occurs commonly with neomycin and bacitracin. Chloramphenicol and sulphonamides from ophthalmic preparations can also cause dermatitis around the eyes. Penicillin is a potent sensitiser so is not used for topical treatment.

Drugs used *systemically* can cause a localised fixed drug eruption or a more diffuse macular or papular erythema, symmetrically distributed. In the later stages exfoliation, with shedding scales of skin, may develop. Antibiotics, particularly penicillins, are the most common cause. They also cause erythema multiforme as already mentioned.

Penicillins are the most common cause of drug rashes, which range from acute anaphylaxis to persistent diffuse erythematous lesions. Joint pains, fever, and proteinuria may be associated, as in serum sickness.

Ampicillin often produces a characteristic erythematous maculopapular rash on the limbs 7–20 days after the start of treatment. Such rashes occur in nearly all patients with infectious mononucleosis who are given ampicillin.

Other reactions

Blistering eruptions	Barbiturates Sulphonamides Iodines/bromides Chlorpropamide Salicylates Phenylbutazone
Lichen planus like reactions	Chloroquine Chlorothiazide Chlorpropamide
Photosensitivity (seen on areas exposed to light)	Thiazide diuretics Sulphonamides Tetracyclines

Topical neomycin allergy.　After withdrawing neomycin.

Vasculitis

Vasculitis

Inflammation around dilated capillaries and small blood vessels:
- a common component of the erythemas
- may occur as red macules and papules with necrotic lesions on the extremities
- in children a purpuric type (Henoch-Schönlein purpura) occurs in association with nephritis
- systemic lesions may occur, with renal, joint, gastrointestinal, and central nervous system involvement.

Inflammation associated with immune complexes in the capillaries and small blood vessels is part of the pathological changes of many of the conditions described above. The term vasculitis is also used clinically to describe a variable clinical picture with red macules and papules and with necrosis and bruising in severe cases. In children purpura is more prominent and these cases are classified as Henoch-Schönlein purpura. The legs and arms are usually affected. Skin signs are preceded by malaise and fever with arthropathy and there may be associated urticaria. Since a high proportion of cases are associated with systemic lesions it is essential to check for renal, joint, gastrointestinal, and central nervous system disease. In children with Henoch-Schönlein purpura nephritis is common.

Purpura

Is seen on the skin as a result of:
- thrombocytopenia—platelet deficiency
- senile purpura—due to shearing of capillaries as a result of defective supporting connective tissue
- purpura in patients on corticosteroid treatment—similar to senile purpura
- Schamberg's disease—brown macules and red spots resembling cayenne pepper on the legs of men
- associated vasculitis.

Acute vasculitis with necrosis.

Some conditions associated with vasculitis

Infection—streptococcal, hepatitis

Drugs—numerous, including sulphonamides, penicillin, phenothiazine, phenacitin

Chemicals—insecticides, weed killers, phenolic compounds

Connective tissue diseases—systemic lupus erythematosus, rheumatoid arthritis

Lymphoma and leukaemia

Dysproteinaemias

Urticaria

Urticaria.

Angio-oedema.

Dermatographism.

In this condition itching red weals develop; they resemble the effects of stinging nettle (*Urtica Dioica*) on the skin. The condition may be associated with allergic reactions, infection, or physical stimuli, but in most patients no cause can be found. Similar lesions may precede, or be associated with, vasculitis (*urticarial vasculitis*), pemphigoid, or dermatitis herpetiformis.

The histological changes may be very slight but usually there is oedema, vasodilation, and a cellular infiltrate of lymphocytes, polymorphs, and histiocytes. Various vasoactive substances are thought to be involved, including histamine, kinins, leukotrienes, prostaglandins, and complement.

Angio-oedema is due to oedema of the subcutaneous tissues; it can occur rapidly and may involve the mucous membranes. *Hereditary angio-oedema* is a rare form with recurrent severe episodes of subcutaneous oedema, swelling of the mucous membranes, and systemic symptoms. Laryngeal oedema is the most serious complication.

The physical uritcarias, which account for about 25% of cases, include *dermatographism* and the *pressure, cold, heat, solar, cholinergic,* and *aquagenic urticarias*.

Dermatographism is an exaggerated release of histamine from stroking the skin firmly with a hard object, such as the end of a pencil. *Pressure urticaria* is caused by sustained pressure from clothing, hard seats, and footwear; it may last some hours. *Cold urticaria* varies in severity and is induced by cold, particularly by cold winds or by the severe shock of bathing in cold water. It appears early in life—in infancy in the rare familial form. In a few cases abnormal serum proteins may be found. *Heat urticaria* is rare, but warm environments often make physical urticaria worse. *Solar urticaria* is a rare condition in which sunlight causes an acute urticarial eruption. Tolerance to sun exposure may develop in areas of the body normally exposed to sun. There is sensitivity to a wide spectrum of ultraviolet light. *Cholinergic urticaria* is characterised by the onset of itching urticarial papules after exertion, stress, or exposure to heat. The injection of cholinergic drugs induces similar lesions in some patients. *Aquagenic urticaria* occurs on contact with water, regardless of the temperature.

Non-physical urticaria may be *acute* in association with allergic reactions to insect bites, drugs, and other factors. Chronic recurrent urticaria is fairly common. Innumerable causes have been suggested but, to the frustration of patient and doctor alike, it is often impossible to identify any specific factor. Some reported causes are listed below.

Some reported causes of non-physical urticaria

Food allergies—fish, eggs, dairy products, chocolate, nuts, strawberries, pork, tomatoes

Food additives—for example, tartrazine dyes, sodium benzoates

Salicylates—both in medicines and foods

Infection—bacterial, viral, and protozoal

Systemic disorders—autoimmune and "collagen" diseases; reticuloses, carcinoma, and dysproteinaemias

Contact urticaria—may occur from contact with meat, fish, vegetables, plants, and animals, among many other factors

Papular urticaria—a term used for persistent itching papules at the site of insect bites; it is also sometimes applied to urticaria from other causes

Inhalants—for example, house dust, animal danders

Treatment

(1) Eliminate possible causative factors, such as aspirin, and by a diet free from food additives.

(2) Antihistamines. Also, H_2 blockers—for example, cimetidine.

(3) Adrenaline can be used for acute attacks, particularly if there is angio-oedema of the respiratory tract.

(4) Systemic corticosteroids should not be used for chronic urticaria but may be needed for acute urticarial vasculitis.

BLISTERS AND PUSTULES

Development, duration, and distribution

The differential diagnosis of blistering eruptions

Widespread blisters

Eczema—Lichenfication and crusting, itching

Dermatitis herpetiformis—Itching, extensor surface, persistent

Chickenpox—Crops of blisters, self limiting, prodromal illness

Pityriasis lichenoides—pink papules, developing blisters

Erythema multiforme—erythematous and "target" lesions, mucous membranes affected

Pemphigoid—Older patients, trunk and flexures affected. Preceding erythematous lesions, deeply situated, tense blisters

Pemphigus—Adults, widespread superficial blisters, mucous membranes affected (erosions)

Drug eruptions—History of drugs prescribed, overdose (barbiturates, tranquillisers)

Localised blisters

Eczema—"Pompholyx" blisters on hand and feet, itching

Allergic reactions, including topical medication, insect bites

Psoriasis—Deep, sterile, non-itching blisters on palms and soles

Impetigo—Usually localised, staphylococci and streptococci isolated

Herpes simplex—Itching lesions developing turbid blisters

Itching	Non-itching	
Eczema-pompholyx on hands and feet	Erythema multiforme	Pustular psoriasis of hands and feet
Allergic reactions	Pemphigus vulgaris	
Dermatitis herpetiformis	Bullous pemphigoid	
Chickenpox	Bullous impetigo	
Herpes simplex	Insect bite allergy	

Several diseases may present with blisters or pustules. There is no common condition that can be used as a "reference point" with which less usual lesions can be compared in the same way as rashes can be compared with psoriasis. A different approach is needed for the assessment of blistering or pustular lesions, based on the history and appearance and summarised as the three Ds: development, duration, and distribution.

Development—Was there any preceding systemic illness—as in chickenpox, hand, foot, and mouth disease, and other viral infections? Was there a preceding area of erythema—as in herpes simplex or pemphigoid? Is the appearance of the lesions associated with itching—as in herpes simplex, dermatitis herpetiformis, and eczematous vesicles on the hands and feet?

Duration—Some acute blistering arises rapidly—for example, in allergic reactions, impetigo, erythema multiforme, and pemphigus. Other blisters have a more gradual onset and follow a chronic course—as in dermatitis herpetiformis, pityriasis lichenoides, and the bullae of porphyria cutanea tarda. The rare genetic disorder epidemolysis bullosa is present from, or soon after, birth.

Distribution—The distribution of blistering rashes helps considerably in making a clinical diagnosis. The most common patterns of those that have a fairly constant distribution are shown.

Itching is a very useful symptom. If all the accessible lesions are scratched and it is hard to find an intact blister it is probably an itching rash.

Clinical features: widespread blisters

Chickenpox

Chickenpox is so well known in general practice that it is rarely seen in hospital clinics and is sometimes not recognised. The prodromal illness lasts one to two days and is followed by erythematous lesions that rapidly develop vesicles, then pustules, followed by crusts in two to three days. Crops of lesions develop at the same sites—usually on the trunk, face, scalp, and limbs. The oral mucosa may be affected. The condition is usually benign.

Dermatitis herpetiformis

Dermatitis herpetiformis occurs in early and middle adult life and is characterised by symmetrical, intensely itching vesicles on the trunk and extensor surfaces. The vesicles are superficial. The onset is gradual, but may occur rapidly. The distribution is shown in the diagram on the next page.

Dermatitis herpetiformis.

Blisters and pustules

Dermatitis herpetiformis.

Erythema multiforme.

Pityriasis lichenoides.

Bullous pemphigoid.

Mucous membrane pemphigoid.

Variants of dematitis herpetiformis are larger blisters forming bullae and erythematous papules and vesicles.

Associated conditions—Coeliac disease with villous atrophy and gluten intolerance may occur in association with dermatitis herpetiformis. Linear IgA disease is a more severe, widespread disease, in which there are "linear" deposits of IgA along the basement membrane of the epidermis and not only at the tips of the papillae as in dermatitis herpetiformis. Treatment is with dapsone or sulphapyridine together with a gluten free diet.

Erythrema multiforme with blisters

Blisters can occur on the lesions of erythema multiforme to a variable degree; when severe, generalised, and affecting the mucous membranes it is known as Stevens Johnson syndrome. The typical erythematous maculopapular changes develop over one to two days with a large blister (bulla) developing in the centre of the target lesions. In severe progressive cases there is extensive disease of the mouth, eyes, genitalia, and respiratory tract. The blisters are subepidermal— that is, deep—although some basement membrane remains on the floor of the blister.

Pityriasis lichenoides varioliformis acuta

As the name implies lichenified papules are the main feature of pityriasis lichenoides varioliformis acuta (or Mucha-Habermann's disease), but vesicles occur in the acute form. Crops of pink papules develop centrally, with vesicles, necrosis, and scales—resembling those of chickenpox, hence the "varioliformis." There is considerable variation in the clinical picture, and a prodromal illness may occur. The condition may last from six weeks to six months. No infective agent has been isolated. The pathological changes parallel the clinical appearance with inflammation around the blood vessels and oedema within the dermis.

Pemphigoid

The bullous type of pemphigoid is a disease of the elderly in which tense bullae develop rapidly, often over a preceding erythematous rash, as well as on normal skin. The flexuaral aspects of the limbs and trunk are mainly affected. The bullae are subepidermal and persistent, with antibodies deposited at the dermoepidermal junction. Unlike pemphigus, there is a tendency for the condition to remit after many months. Treatment is with corticosteroids by mouth, 40 to 60 mg daily in most patients, although higher doses are required by some. Azathioprine aids remission, with reduced steroid requirements, but takes some weeks to produce an effect. Topical steroids can be used on developing lesions.

Chronic scarring pemphigoid affects the mucous membranes with small bullae that break down, leading to erosions and adhesions in the conjunctivae, mouth, pharynx, and genitalia.

There is also a localised type of pemphigoid occurring on the legs of elderly women that runs a benign self limiting course.

32

Blisters and pustules

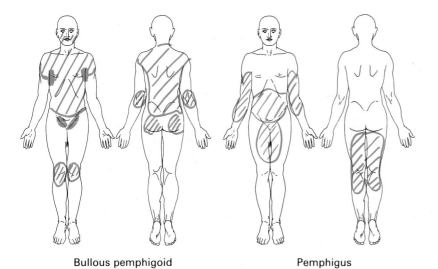

Bullous pemphigoid   Pemphigus

Pemphigus

The most common form of pemphigus vulgaris is a chronic progressive condition with widespread superficial bullae arising in normal skin. In about half of the cases this is preceded by blisters and erosions in the mouth. The bullae are easily broken, and even rubbing apparently normal skin causes the superficial epidermis to slough off (Nikolsky sign). These changes are associated with the deposition of immunoglobulin in the epidermal intercellular spaces. It is a serious condition with high morbidity despite treatment with steroids and azathioprine.

Pemphigus vegetans and pemphigus erythematosus are less common variants.

Pemphigus vulgaris.

Nikolsky sign.

Ulcers in the mouth

Differential diagnosis:

Trauma (dentures)

Aphthous ulcers

Candida albicans infection

Herpes simplex

Erythema multiforme (from drugs)

Pemphigus

Lichen planus

Carcinoma

Clinical features: localised blisters

Pompholyx—which means "a bubble"—is characterised by persistent, itchy, clear blisters on the fingers, which may extend to the palms, with larger blisters. The feet may be affected. Secondary infection leads to turbid vesicle fluid. Pompholyx may be associated with a number of conditions—atopy, stress, fungal infection elsewhere, and allergic reactions. It may occur as a result of ingesting nickel in nickel sensitive patients and a similar reaction has been reported to neomycin.

Pustular psoriasis is characterised by deep seated sterile blisters, often with no sign of psoriasis elsewhere—hence the term *palmopustular pustulosis*. Foci of sepsis have long been considered a causative factor and recent studies have shown a definite association with cigarette smoking. The pattern of HLA antigens indicates that this may be a separate condition from psoriasis.

Blisters and pustules

Bullous impetigo is seen in children and adults. Staphylococci are usually isolated from the blister fluid. The blisters are commonly seen on the face and are more deeply situated than in the non-bullous variety.

Herpes simplex—Primary infection with type I virus occurs on the face, lips, and buccal mucosa in children and young adults. Type II viruses cause genital infection. Itching may be severe.

Herpes zoster is due to varicella virus producing groups of vesicles in a dermatome distribution, usually thoracic, trigeminal, or lumbosacral. It is more common after the fourth decade of life.

Insect bite allergy—Large blisters, which are usually not itching, can occur on the legs of susceptible individuals.

Insect bite allergy.   Drug reaction to sulphapyridine.

Bullous drug eruptions

Fixed drug eruptions can develop bullae, and some drugs can cause a generalised bullous eruption, particularly:
- Barbiturates (particularly if taken in overdosage)
- Sulphonamides
- Penicillamine (captopril, penicillins (which produce pemphigus-like bullae))
- Frusemide (may be phototoxic)

Remember that there may be an associated erythematous eruption.

LEG ULCERS

Although the patient will not probably die of this disease, yet, without great care, it may render her miserable. The disease may be very much relieved by art, and it is one of very common occurrence.

SIR BENJAMIN BRODIE (1846)

Despite the great increase in our understanding of the pathology of leg ulcers, their management is still largely "art." Consequently there are numerous treatments, each with their enthusiastic advocates. There are, however, basic concepts which are helpful in management. Since about 95% of leg ulcers are of the "venous" or gravitational variety these will be considered first.

Pathology of venous ulcers

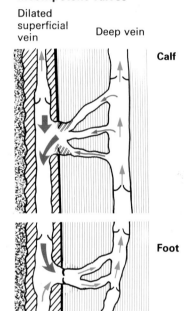

Healthy

Superficial vein
Deep vein
Calf

Skin | Rigid Muscle "pump"
fascia

Subcutaneous tissue

Incompetent valves

Dilated superficial vein
Deep vein
Calf

Foot

Varicose veins.   Ulcers and fibrosis.

The skin—Ulcers arise because the skin dies from inadequate provision of nutrients and oxygen. This occurs as a consequence of (*a*) oedema in the subcutaneous tissues with poor lymphatic and capillary drainage; and (*b*) the extravascular accumulation of fibrinous material that has leaked from the blood vessels. The result is a rigid cuff around the capillaries, preventing diffusion through the wall, and fibrosis of the surrounding tissues.

The blood vessels—Arterial perfusion of the leg is usually normal or increased, but stasis occurs in the venules. The lack of venous drainage is a consquence of incompetent valves between the superficial veins and the deeper large veins on which the calf muscle "pump" acts. In the norml leg there is a *superficial* low pressure venous system and *deep* high pressure veins. If the blood flow from superficial to deep veins is reversed then the pressure in the superficial veins may increase to a level that prevents venous drainage with "back pressure" causing stasis and oedema.

Incompetent valves leading to gravitational ulcers may be preceded by:

(*a*) deep vein thrombosis associated with pregnancy or, less commonly, leg injury, immobilisation, or infarctions in the past;

(*b*) primary long saphenous vein insufficiency;

(*c*) familial venous valve incompetence that presents at an earlier stage. There is a familial predisposition in half of all patients with leg ulcers; or

(*d*) deep venous obstruction.

Who gets ulcers?

Mainly women get ulcers—2% of those over 80 having venous ulcers as a long term consequence of the factors listed above. Leg ulcers are more likely to occur and are more severe in obese people.

Clinical changes

Atrophie blanche.

Champagne bottle legs.

Oedema and fibrinous exudate often lead to fibrosis of the subcutaneous tissues, which may be associated with localised loss of pigment and dilated capillary loops, an appearance known as "atrophie blanche." This occurs around the ankle with oedema and dilated tortuous superficial veins proximally and can lead to "champagne bottle legs," the bottle, of course, being inverted. Ulceration often occurs for the first time after a trivial injury.

Lymphoedema results from obliteration of the superficial lymphatics, with associated fibrosis. There is often hypertrophy of the overlying epidermis with a "polypoid" appearance, also known as lipodermatosclerosis.

Venous ulcers occur around the ankles, commonly over the medial malleolus. The margin is usually well defined with a shelving edge, and a slough may be present. There may also be surrounding eczematous changes. Venous ulcers are not usually painful but arterial ulcers are.

It is important to check the pulses in the leg and foot as compression bandaging of a leg with impaired blood flow can cause ischaemia and necrosis.

Treatment

When new epidermis can grow across an ulcer it will and the aim is to produce an environment in which this can take place. To this end several measures can be taken.

(1) *Oedema* may be reduced by means of (*a*) diuretics, (*b*) keeping the legs elevated when sitting, (*c*) avoiding standing as far as possible. Raising the heels slightly from time to time helps venous return by the "calf muscle pump," (*d*) applying compression bandages, which may do more harm than good *unless* they are applied *before* the patient gets out of bed in the morning, when there is minimal oedema, and applied with more pressure on the foot than the calf, so as to create a pressure gradient towards the thigh.

(2) *Exudate and slough* should be removed. Lotions can be used to clean the ulcer and as compresses—0·9% saline solution, sodium hypochlorite solution, Eusol, or 5% hydrogen peroxide.

There is some evidence that antiseptic solutions and chlorinated solutions (such as sodium hypochlorite and Eusol) delay collagen production and cause inflammation. Enzyme preparations may help by "digesting" the slough. To prevent the formation of granulation tissue use silver nitrate 0·25% compresses, a silver nitrate "stick" for more exuberant tissue, and curettage, if necessary.

(3) *The dressings* applied to the ulcer can consist of (*a*) simple non-stick, paraffin gauze dressings. An allergy may develop to those with an antibiotic; (*b*) wet compresses with saline or silver nitrate solutions for exudative lesions; (*c*) silver sulphadiazine (Flamazine) or hydrogen peroxide creams (Hioxyl); and (*d*) absorbent dressings, consisting of hydrocolloid patches or powder, which are helpful for smaller ulcers.

(4) *Paste bandages*, impregnated with zinc oxide and antiseptics or ichthammol, help to keep dressings in place and provide protection. They may, however, traumatise the skin, and allergic reactions to their constituents are not uncommon.

(5) *Treatment of infection* is less often necessary than is commonly supposed. All ulcers are colonised by bacteria to some extent, usually coincidental staphylococci. A purulent exudate is an indication for a broad spectrum antibiotic and a swab for bacteriology. Erythema, oedema, and tenderness around the ulcers suggest a β haemolytic streptococcal infection, which will require long term antibiotic treatment. Dyes can be painted on the edge of the ulcer, where they fix to the bacterial wall as well as the patient's skin. In Scotland bright red eosin is traditionally used, while in the south a blue dye, gentian violet, is favoured.

Systemic antibiotics have little effect on ulcers but are indicated if there is surrounding cellulitis. A swab for culture and sensitivity helps to keep track of organisms colonising the area.

(6) *Surrounding eczematous changes* should be treated. Use topical steroids, not more than medium strength, avoiding the ulcer itself. Ichthammol 1% in 15% zinc oxide and white soft paraffin or Ichthopaste bandages can be used as a protective layer, and topical antibiotics can be used if necessary. It is important to remember that any of the commonly used topical preparations can cause an allergic reaction: neomycin, lanolin, formaldehyde, tars, Clinaform (the "C" of many proprietary steroids).

(7) *Skin grafting* can be very effective. There must be a healthy viable base for the graft, with an adequate blood supply; natural re-epithelialisation from the edges of the ulcer is a good indication that a graft will be supported. Pinch grafts or partial thickness grafts can be used. Any clinical infection, particularly with pseudomonal organisms, should be treated.

(8) *Maintaining general health*, with adequate nutrition and weight reduction, is important.

(9) *Corrective surgery* for associated venous abnormalities.

In treating venous leg ulcers
(1) Take measures to eliminate oedema and reduce weight—make sure the patient understands these.
(2) Never apply steroid preparations to the ulcer itself or it will not heal. Make sure that both nurses and patients are aware of this.
(3) Beware of allergy developing to topical agents—especially to antibiotics.

(4) There is no need to submit the patient to a variety of antibiotics according to the differing bacteria isolated from leg ulcer slough, unless there is definite evidence of infection of adjacent tissue clinically.
(5) A vascular "flare" round the ankle and heel with varicose veins, sclerosis, or oedema indicates a high risk of ulceration developing.
(6) Make sure arterial pulses are present.

Arterial ulcers

Ulcers on the leg also occur as a result of (*a*) atherosclerosis with poor peripheral circulation, particularly in older patients: (*b*) vasculitis affecting the larger subcutaneous arteries; and (*c*) aterial obstruction in macroglobulinaemia, cryoglobulinaemia, polycythaemia, and "collagen" disease—particularly rheumatoid arthritis.

Arterial ulcers are sharply defined and accompanied by pain, which may be very severe, especially at night. The leg, especially the pretibial area, is affected rather than the ankle. In patients with hypertension a very tender ulcer can develop posteriorly (Martorelli's ulcer).

As mentioned above, compression bandaging will make arterial ulcers worse and may lead to ischaemia of the leg.

Diagnosis

The differing presentation of arterial and venous ulcers helps in distinguishing between them, but some degree of aterial insufficiency often complicates venous ulcers.

Phlebography and Doppler ultrasound may help in detecting venous incompetence and arterial obstruction, which can sometimes be treated surgically.

Ulcers on the leg may also occur secondary to other diseases, because of infection, in malignant disease, and after trauma.

Secondary ulcers—Ulcers occur in diabetes, in periarteritis nodosa, and in vasculitis. Pyoderma gangrenosum, a chronic necrotic ulcer with surrounding induration, may occur in association with ulcerative colitis or rheumatoid vasculitis.

Ulcer in diabetic foot.

Leg ulcers

Squamous cell carcinoma in venous ulcer. Tuberculous ulceration.

Infections that cause ulcers include staphylococcal or streptococcal infections, tuberculosis (which is rare in the United Kingdom but may be seen in recent immigrants), and anthrax.

Malignant diseases—Squamous cell carcinoma may present as an ulcer or, rarely, develop in a pre-existing ulcer. Basal cell carcinoma and melanoma may develop into ulcers, as may Kaposi's sarcoma.

Dermatitis artefacta.

Trauma—Patients with diabetic or other types of neuropathy are at risk of developing trophic ulcers. Rarely they may be self induced—"dermatitis artefacta."

ACNE AND ROSACEA

Acne goes with adolescence, a term derived from the Greek "acme" or prime of life. The young girl who is desperately aware of the smallest comedo and the otherwise handsome young man, with his face or back a battle field of acne cysts and scars, are familiar to us all. Both need treatment.

What is acne?

Acne lesions develop from the sebaceous glands associated with hair follicles—on the face, external auditory meatus, back, chest, and anogenital area. Sebaceous glands are also found on the eyelids and mucosa, prepuce and cervix, where they are not associated with hair follicles.) The sebaceous gland contains holocrine cells that secrete triglycerides, fatty acids, wax esters, and sterols as "sebum." The main changes in acne are:

(*a*) an increase in sebum secretion;
(*b*) thickening of the keratin lining of the sebaceous duct, to produce blackheads or comedones. The colour of blackheads is due to melanin, not dirt;
(*c*) an increase in *Propionibacterium acnes* bacteria in the duct;
(*d*) an increase in free fatty acids;
(*e*) inflammation around the sebaceous gland; probably as a result of the release of bacterial enzymes.

Underlying causes

There are various underlying causes of these changes.
Hormones—Androgenic hormones increase the size of sebaceous glands and the amount of sebum in both male and female adolescents. Oestrogens have the opposite effect in prepubertal boys and eunuchs. In some women with acne there is lowering of the concentration of sex hormone binding globulin and a consequent increase in free testosterone concentrations. There is probably also a variable increase in androgen sensitivity. Oral contraceptives containing more than 50 µg ethinyloestradiol can make acne worse and the combined type may lower sex hormone binding globulin concentrations, leading to increased free testosterone. Infantile acne occurs in the first few months of life and may last some years. Apart from rare causes, such as adrenal hyperplasia or virilising tumours, transplacental simulation of the adrenal gland is thought to result in the release of adrenal androgens—but this does not explain why the lesions persist. It is more common in boys.
Fluid retention—The premenstrual exacerbation of acne is thought to be due to fluid retention leading to increased hydration of and swelling of the duct. Sweating also makes acne worse, possibly by the same mechanism.

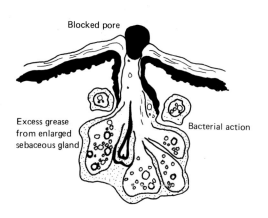

Blocked pore

Excess grease from enlarged sebaceous gland

Bacterial action

Diet—in some patients acne is made worse by chocolate, nuts, and coffee or fizzy drinks.

Seasons—Acne often improves with natural sunlight and is worse in winter. The effect of artificial ultraviolet light is unpredictable.

External factors—Oils, whether vegetable oils in the case of cooks in hot kitchens or mineral oils in engineering, can cause "oil folliculitis," leading to acne like lesions. Other acnegenic substances include coal tar, dicophane (DDT), cutting oils, and halogenated hydrocarbons (polychlorinated biphenols and related chemicals). Cosmetic acne is seen in adult women who have used cosmetics containing comedogenic oils over many years.

Iatrogenic—Corticosteroids, both topical and systemic, can cause increased keratinisation of the pilosebaceous duct. Androgens, gonadotrophins, and corticotrophin can induce acne in adolescence. Oral contraceptives of the combined type can induce acne, and antiepileptic drugs are reputed to cause acne.

Hormones—the cause of all the trouble

Androgens	increase the size of sebaceous glands
	increase sebum secretion
Androgenic adrenocorticosteroids have the same effect	
Ostrogens	have the opposite effect

Types of acne

Acne keloidalis.

Acne vulgaris

Acne vulgaris, the common type of acne, occurs during puberty and affects the comedogenic areas of the face, back, and chest. There may be a familial tendency to acne. Acne vulgaris is slightly more common in boys, 30–40% of whom have acne between the ages of 18 and 19. In girls the peak incidence is between 16 and 18 years. Adult acne is a variant, affecting 1% of men and 5% of women aged 40. Acne keloidalis is a type of scarring acne seen on the neck in men.

Patients with acne often complain of excessive greasiness of the skin, with "blackheads," "pimples," or "plukes" developing. These may be associated with inflammatory papules and pustules developing into larger cysts and nodules. Resolving lesions leave inflammatory macules and scarring. Scars may be atrophic, sometimes with "ice pick" lesions or keloid formation. Keloids consist of hypertrophic scar tissue and occur predominantly on the neck, upper back, and shoulders and over the sternum.

Infantile acne—Localised acne lesions occur on the face in the first few months of life. They clear spontaneously but may last for some years. There is said to be an associated increased tendency to severe adolescent acne.

Acne conglobata. Acne fulminans. Pyoderma faciale.

Acne conglobata—This is a severe form of acne, more common in boys and in tropical climates. It is extensive, affecting the trunk, face, and limbs. In "acne fulminans" there is associated systemic illness with malaise, fever, and joint pains. It appears to be associated with a hypersensitivity to *P acnes*. Another variant is pyoderma faciale, which produces erythematous and necrotic lesions and occurs mainly in adult women.

Acne vulgaris

   affects comedogenic areas
   occurs mainly in puberty,
      in boys more than girls
   familial tendency

Infantile acne

   face only
   clears spontaneously

Severe acne

   acne conglobata
   pyoderma faciale
   Gram negative folliculitis

Occupational acne

   oils
   coal and tar
   chlorinated phenols
   DDT and weedkillers

Steroids

   systemic or topical

Acne vulgaris.

Hormones

   combined type of oral
   contraceptives and
   androgenic hormones

Gram negative folliculitis.

Gram negative folliculitis occurs with a proliferation of organisms such as klebsiella, proteus, pseudomonas, and *Escherichia coli.*

Occupatonal—Acne like lesions occur as a result of long term contact with oils or tar as mentioned above. This usually occurs as a result of lubricating, cutting, or crude oil soaking through clothing. In chloracne there are prominent comedones on the face and neck. It is caused by exposure to polychlortriphenyl and related compounds and also to weedkiller and dicophane.

Treatment of acne

Before and after treatment with tetracycline.

In most adolescents acne clears spontaneously with minimal scarring. Reassurance and explanation along the following lines helps greatly.

(1) The lesions can be expected to clear in time.
(2) It is not infectious.
(3) The less sufferers are self conscious and worry about their appearance the less other people will take any notice of their acne.

It helps to give a simple regimen to follow, enabling patients to take some positive steps to clear their skin and also an alternative to picking their spots.

I advise patients with acne to hold a hot wet flannel on the face (a much simpler alternative to the commercial "facial saunas"), followed by gentle rubbing in of a plain soap. Savlon solution, diluted 10 times with water, is an excellent alternative for controlling greasy skin.

There are many proprietary preparations, most of which act as keratolytics, dissolving the keratin plug of the comedone. They can also cause considerable dryness and scaling of the skin.

Benzoyl peroxide in concentrations of 1% to 10% comes as lotions, creams, gels, and washes. Resorcinol, sulphur, and salicylic acid preparations are also available.

Vitamin A acid as a cream or gel is helpful in some patients. A topical retinal gel has recently been introduced.

Ultraviolet light therapy is less effective than natural sunlight but is helpful for extensive acne.

Oral treatment—The mainstay of treatment is oxytetracycline, which should be given for a week at 1 g daily then 500 mg (250 mg twice daily) on an empty stomach. Minocycline or doxycycline are alternatives that can be taken with food. Perseverance with treatment is important, and it may take some months to produce an appreciable improvement. Erythromycin is an alternative to tetracycline, and co-trimoxazole can be used for Gram negative folliculitis. Tetracycline might theoretically interfere with the action of progesterone types of birth control pill and should not be given in pregnancy.

Topical antibiotics—Erythromycin, the tetracyclines, and clindamycin have been used topically. There is the risk of producing colonies of resistant organisms.

Acne and rosacea

Before and after treatment with ultravioet light.

Antiandrogens—Cyproterone acetate combined with ethinyloestradiol is effective in some women; it is also a contraceptive.

Synthetic retinoids—For severe cases resistant to other treatments these drugs, which can be prescribed only in hospital, are very effective and clear most cases in a few months. 13-*cis*-Retinoic acid (isotretinoin) is usually used for acne. They are teratogenic, so there must be no question of pregnancy, and can cause liver changes with raised serum lipid values. Regular blood tests are therefore essential. A three month course of treatment usually gives a long remission. Recently topical isotretinoin gel has been introduced.

Ultraviolet light is a helpful additional treatment in the winter months.

Keloid scars.

Keloid scars on dark skin.

Residual lesions, keloid scars, cysts, and persistent nodules can be treated by injection with triamcinolone or freezing with liquid nitrogen. For severe scarring dermabrasion can produce good cosmetic results. This is usually carried out in a plastic surgery unit.

Remember the following points

(1) Avoid topical steroids
(2) Persevere with one antibiotic not short courses of different types
(3) Do not prescribe a tetracycline for children and pregnant women
(4) Oxytetracycline must be taken on an empty stomach half an hour before meals

Treatment of acne

First line

(1) Encourage positive attitudes
(2) Avoid environmental and occupational factors
(3) Topical treatment
   Benzoyl peroxide
   Salicylic acid
(4) A tetracycline by mouth for several months

Second line

(1) Topical vitamin A acid
(2) Topical antibiotics
(3) Ultraviolet light
(4) Antiandrogens

Third line

Oral retinoids for 3–4 months (hospitals only)

Rosacea

Blepharitis.

Rosacea is a persistent eruption occurring on the forehead and cheeks. It is more common in women than men.

There is erythema with prominent blood vessels. Pustules, papules, and oedema occur. Rhinophyma, with thickened erythematous skin of the nose and enlarged follicles, is a variant. Conjunctivitis and blepharitis may be associated. It is usually made worse by sunlight.

Rosacea.

Rosacea.

Rosacea.

Rhinophyma.

Lupus erythematosus.

Perioral dermatitis.

Rosacea should be distinguished from:

Acne, in which there are blackheads, a wider distribution, and improvement with sunlight. Acne, however, may coexist with rosacea—hence the older term "acne rosacea";

Seborrhoeic eczema, in which there are no pustules and eczematous changes are present;

Lupus erythematosus, which shows light sensitivity, erythema, and scarring but no pustules;

Perioral dermatitis, which occurs in women with pustules and erythema around the mouth and on the chin. There is usually a premenstrual exacerbation. Treatment is with oral tetracyclines.

Treatment

The treatment of rosacea is with long term courses of oxytetracycline, which may need to be repeated. Topical treatment along the lines of that for acne is also helpful. Topical steroids should not be used as they have minimal effect and cause a severe rebound erythema, which is difficult to clear. Avoiding hot and spicy foods may help.

Recent reports indicate that synthetic retinoids are also effective.

BACTERIAL INFECTION

The process of infection involves the interaction of two organisms—host and invader. The clinical changes are a manifestation of the resulting "battle of the cells" as so clearly perceived by Metchnikoff 100 years ago. The lesions produced may have a well recognised appearance, such as impetigo or tinea cruris, but are often less specific.

Several features enable us to recognise that infection is a possible cause of the patient's condition.

Acute bacterial infections produce the classical characteristics of acute inflammation described by Celsus (see box).

Presentation

Presentation.

Two weeks later.

This woman had acute *erysipelas* due to haemolytic streptococcus, and all four features were present. She was, however, referred to the clinic with a diagnosis of acute allergy, which, from the appearance alone, was understandable. However, malaise and fever were also present and the lesions were warm. The condition responded well to antibiotic treatment. The point of entry in such cases may be a "spot" on the face or a small erosion near the nose, mouth, or ears. Erysipelas of the leg or foot may follow a small fissure between the toes.

Erysipelas is the local manifestation of a streptococcal infection, but this organism in the throat can result in the widespread rash of scarlet fever, which is rarely seen these days, or erythema multiforme, which is more common. An acute generalised vasculitis can also be associated with a streptococcal infection.

(1) In any patient with a localised area of acute erythema, swelling, and raised temperature consider infection.

(2) Remember that a *generalised* erythematous rash may be the manifestation of a *localised* infection. Scarlet fever arises from streptococcal throat infection, and herpes simplex of the lip may be associated with erythema multiforme.

(3) The common pathogens are also commensals—recent studies showed that 60% of individuals are nasal carriers of *Staphylococcus aureus* intermittently and 10% carry *Streptococcus pyogenes* in the throat.

More chronic forms of bacterial infection include *impetigo, folliculitis, carbuncles,* and *ecthyma*. These conditions are due to streptococci and particularly to staphylococci, which are adept at colonising the skin, commonly in those with atopic eczema. Bacterial infection occurs in eczematous lesions and may itself cause an exacerbation of eczema.

Impetigo is a superficial infection of the skin, with transient blisters in the non-bullous form that then form crusts. Both staphylococci and streptococci are responsible. The bullous form is due to staphylococci.

Folliculitis, with infection and inflammatory changes in the upper follicle, is common. Deeper forms occur in the scalp (follicular impetigo) or the beard area (sycosis barbae). Abscess formation in the hair follicles results in furuncles or boils; several may coalesce to form a carbuncle.

Ecthyma, which is most common on the leg, is due to bacterial infection causing a necrotic lesion with a superficial crust and surrounding inflammation. Both streptococci and staphylococci are responsible.

Mycobacterial disease

Lupus vulgaris.

Swimming pool granuloma.

Tuberculoid leprosy.

The clinical presentation of mycobaceterial disease depends on the immune response of the host—hence the difference between disseminated miliary tuberculosis and lupus vulgaris or, for example, tuberculoid and lepromatous leprosy.

These infections are rarely seen in the West so only the most common types—lupus vulgaris and "atypical mycobacterial infection" are described.

Lupus vulgaris is a very slowly growing indolent condition of the skin. The lesion shown had been present for 20 years and may have been acquired from the cattle with which the man worked. The characteristic giant cell granuloma can be clearly seen.

Atypical mycobacterial infections—Although infection with *Mycobacterium tuberculosis* is now rare in Britain, other types of mycobacterial skin infection occur. The most common is "fishtank" or "swimming pool" granuloma, aquired from tropical fish tackle or swimming pools, respectively, and caused by *Mycobacterium marinum*. Nodular lesions develop slowly with ulceration but there is no regional lymph node enlargement. *Mycobacterium kansasii* infection is rare and *Mycobacterium ulcerans* confined to the tropics.

Erythema of the face

Acute

	Usually unilateral	Usually bilateral	Photosensitive
(1) Allergic reactions			
Cosmetics (*left*)		+	+ or −
Plants	+	or +	+ or −
Drugs		+	+ or −
(2) Urticaria		+	−
Reactions to light			
(3) Photodermatitis (*right*)		+	+
Solar urticaria		+	+
(4) Infection			
Erysipelas (*left*)		+	−
Fifth disease ("slapped cheek")		+	−
(5) Rosacea (*right*)		+	+ or −

Chronic-recurrent

	Usually unilateral	Usually bilateral	Photosensitive
(6) Lupus erythematosus			
Systemic (*left*)		+	+
Discoid (*right*)	+	or +	+
(7) Seborrhoeic dermatitis (*left*)		+	−
(8) Acne		+	+
(9) Perioral dermatitis (*right*)		+	−

Common patterns of cutaneous bacterial infection

	Infected eczema	*Impetigo (non-bullous)*	*Impetigo (bullous)*
Appearance			
	Exudate Crusts Inflamation	Transient vesicles Exuding lesions with yellow crusts Erythema Affects mainly face and limbs, commonly in children	Erythema and bullae which rupture to leave superficial crusts May be central clearing Affects face, buttocks, and limbs in children and adults
Cause	Persistent scratching Topical steroids	Local reaction between invading organisms and neutrophils, resulting in superficial epidermal split in bullous lesion	
Organism	Staphylococcus arueus Streptococcus pyogenes	Staphylococcus aureus Streptococcus pyogenes in some outbreaks	Staphylococcus aureus
Treatment	(1) Weaker topical steroids (for the eczema) with topical antibiotics (2) Systemic antibiotics if necessary (3) Soaks with potassium permanganate (4) 1% eosin or gentian violet to paint erosions	Topical antibiotics Systemic antibiotics directed against both streptococcal and staphylococcal infection	Topical and systemic antibiotics
Notes	• Avoid prolonged use of topical antibiotics • Return to using weaker steroid when infection has healed • Even without clinical evidence of infection most lesions of atopic eczema are colonised by *Staphylococcus aureus*	• Staphylococcal infection can cause widespread superficial shedding of the epidermis—"scalded skin syndrome" (Lyell's disease) • It is wise to send a specimen for bacteriology: nephritogenic strains of streptococcus in impetigo remain an important cause for glomerulonephritis, although this is a rare condition.	

Boils (and furuncles) and carbuncles	Folliculitis	Ecthyma	Erysipelas
Inflammatory nodule affecting the hair follicles develops into a pustule Tender induration with considerable inflammation, followed by necrosis Heals with scarring More common in adolescents in winter Several boils may coalesce to form a carbuncle	Various forms: (1) *Scalp* Children—"Follicular impetigo" *Adults—* (*a*) Folliculitis cheloidalis Back of neck (*b*) Acne necrotica Forehead/hairline (2) *Face*—"Sycosis barbae" in men with seborrhoea (greasy skin) (3) *Legs*—Chronic folliculitis	Small bullae may be present initially An adherent crust is followed by a purulent ulcerated lesion with surrounding erythema and induration, which slowly heals Usually on legs	Well defined areas of erythema—very tender, not oedematous Vesicles may form Common sites—abdominal wall in infants; in adults the lower leg and face An area of broken skin, forming a portal of entry, may be found
Possible anaemia and fatigue Mechanical damage from clothing	(1) Underlying disease—eg diabetes (2) Infection may be precipitated by mechanical injury, tar pastes, and occlusive dressings	Minor injuries More common in debilitated individuals	Lymphoedema and severe inflammation due to bacterial toxins
Staphylococcus aureus, usually of same strain as in nose and perineum	*Staphylococcus aureus* *Propionibacterium acnes* *Pityrosporum* spp *Pseudomonas* spp and other Gram negative organisms	Both streptococcus and staphylococcus	*Streptococcus pyogenes* (group A, but may be B, C, or G) *Staphylococcus aureus* *Klebsiella pneumoniae* *Haemophilus influenzae*
(1) Antibiotic (penicillinase resistant) systemically (2) Cleaning of skin with weak chlorhexedine solution or a similar preparation	Topical and long term systemic antibiotics—eg oxytetracycline Topical antifungal for pityrosporum infection	Improve nutrition Use antibiotic effective against both staphylococcus and streptococcus	Penicillin or erythromycin

- Nasal and perineal swabs should be taken to identify carriers
- Remember unusual causes—a bricklayer presented with a boil on the arm with necrosis due to anthrax (malignant pustule) acquired from the packing straw used for the bricks

- Gram negative folliculitis occurs on the face—a complication of long term treatment for acne
- A persistent, painful type of necrotic folliculitis occurs in those who wear hats, caps, or helmets for long periods

- Check for debilitating diseases, reticuloses, diabetes

- Cellulitis affects the deeper tissues and has more diverse causes, being essentially inflammation of the connective tissue
- Streptococcus, staphylococcus, haemophilus, and other organisms may be found
- Beware of erysipelas of the face—the venous drainage is deep to the cavernous sinus. A young resident physician decided to "tough out" her erysipelas on the cheek and refused treatment. Severe fever, facial oedema, and malaise associated with cavernous sinus phlebitis followed

VIRAL INFECTIONS

Molluscum inclusion bodies (a pox virus).

Herpes

Herpes of lips.

Inoculation herpes.   Genital herpes.

Eczema herpeticum.   Herpes zoster.

Like the pyogenic bacteria, viruses produce local lesions and may cause a widespread reaction to the infection. The clinical manifestations of common viral infections of the skin are well known and easily recognised.

Local infective lesions are caused by DNA viruses which can be isolated from the lesions themselves and include the herpes and pox groups.

In patients with AIDS florid and widespread viral infections of the skin occur.

Herpes simplex

The herpes simplex virus consists of two antigenic types. Type I is associated with lesions on the face and fingers and sometimes genital lesions. Type II is associated almost entirely with genital infections.

Primary herpes simplex (type I) infection usually occurs in or around the mouth, with variable involvement of the face. Although there is usually a small area of inflammation with irritation forming a vesicle, there may be considerable inflammation and necrosis with malaise, probably depending on the degree of protection from maternal antibodies. Subsequent recurrent chronic infection of the lips may be due to virus remaining in the sensory nerve ganglia.

Type II infection affects the genitalia, vagina, and cervix and may predispose to cervical dysplasia
● The initial vesicular stage may not be seen in genital lesions, which present as painful ulcers or erosions
● There is usually a history of preceding itching and tenderness
● Scrapings from the base of the ulcer can be stained for viral inclusion bodies (Tzanck smears). The virus can often be cultured from vesicle fluid. Viral antigen can be shown by immunofluorescence
● Genital herpes in a pregnant woman carries a great risk of ophthalmic infection of the infant. Caesarean section may be indicated
● "Eczema herpeticum" or "Kaposi's varicelliform eruption" are terms applied to lifethreatening systemic infection with herpes virus in patients with atopic eczema and some other skin conditions. Treatment is with parenteral acyclovir. It can also be caused by vaccinia and coxsackie viruses.

Herpes zoster

Herpes zoster, due to herpesvirus varicella, which also causes chickenpox (due to a herpes virus, not a pox virus), develops without a definable incubation period. There is, however, often pain, fever, and malaise before erythematous papules develop in the area of the affected dermatome—most commonly in the thoracic area. Vesicles develop over several days, leaving dried crusts as they resolve. Secondary infection is common. The subsequent neuralgia, particularly in elderly people, is well known.

● Trigeminal zoster may occur and affect the ophthalmic nerve (causing severe conjunctivitis); the maxillary nerve (causing vesicles on the uvula or tonsils); or the mandibular nerve (causing vesicles on the floor of the mouth and on the tongue)
● Visceral lesions can occur with pleuritic and abdominal pain
● Disseminated zoster is a severe illness, often with haemorrhagic lesions.

48

Mandibular zoster.

Ophthalmic zoster.

Pox viruses

Molluscum contagiosum.

Cowpox, early stage.

Milkers' node.

Remember that infection from both skin lesions and nasopharyngeal secretions can cause chickenpox.

Treatment

The usual troublesome, localised lesions of herpes simplex have been treated with topical zinc sulphate, iodoxuridine, ice cubes, and photoactivation of eosin. Topical acyclovir—a drug that inhibits herpes virus DNA polymerase—is effective and should be used as soon as the patient is aware of symptoms.

Severe, recurrent, herpes simplex or herpes zoster can be treated with acyclovir by mouth or injection, given as early in the course of the illness as possible.

Secondary infection may require antiseptic soaks, such as 1/1000 potassium permanganate, or topical or systemic antibiotics.

Steroids (prednisolone 40–60 mg/day) given during the acute stage of herpes zoster diminish pain and postherpetic neuralgia.

Rest and analgesics are recommended treatment for extensive herpes simplex or herpes zoster infections.

> **Steroids should not be given to immunodeficient patients, in whom they may cause disseminated infection**

The pox viruses are also large DNA viruses, particularly infecting the epidermis.

Variola (smallpox), once the cause of high mortality, has been officially eliminated by vaccination with modified vaccinia virus—the culmination of Jenner's pioneer work.

Molluscum contagiosum

The commonest "pox" seen these days is molluscum contagiosum—a worry to mothers of affected infants, who are not themselves unduly concerned. Despite its name it is not very contagious, except in overcrowded conditions in tropical countries. In temperate climates it often affects only one or two children in a household.

Clinical features—The white, umbilicated papules of molluscum contagiosum are characteristic. Large solitary lesions may cause confusion and so can secondarily infected, excoriated lesions. Remember that these can itch, particularly in patients with atopy. There may be widespread lesions in patients with AIDS and which are said to be more common in sarcoidosis and atopy.

Diagnosis is not difficult. Sometimes there is confusion with viral warts and, in a solitary lesion, benign tumour of the skin.

Treatment—Most treatments are painful and should not be inflicted on a child with a benign self limiting condition. An antibiotic-hydrocortisone ointment can be used for excoriated lesions. Treatment with liquid nitrogen is probably the simplest treatment. Other methods include superficial curettage and carefully rotating a sharpened orange stick moistened with phenol in the centre of each lesion.

Other pox infections

The other pox infections are of incidental interest.

Cowpox only sporadically infects cows from its natural reservoir, probably small mammals, and may affect humans. Papules on the hands enlarge and develop necrosis and crusting.

Milkers' nodules are due to a virus that causes superficial ulcers in cows' udders and calves' mouths. In humans papules form on the hands and develop into grey nodules with a necrotic centre, surrounding inflammation, and lymphangeitis. A more generalised papular eruption can occur.

Orf is easily diagnosed by country doctors, sheep farmers, and veterinarians but may be overinvestigated by those less familiar with rural dermatology. It is seen mainly in early spring as a result of contact with lambs. A single papule or group of lesions develops on the

Viral infections

Orf.

fingers or hands with purple papules developing into a bulla. This ruptures to leave an annular lesion 1–3 cm in diameter with a necrotic centre. There is surrounding inflammation. The incubation period is a few days and the lesions last 2–3 weeks with spontaneous healing. Associated erythema multiforme and widespread rashes are occasionally seen.

Monkey pox, *reindeer pox*, and *musk ox pox* are of interest to those treating zookeepers and travellers.

Wart viruses

Common warts.

The true worth of the papilloma virus, which causes warts, as an object of serious study has only recently been recognised. The wart is, after all, one of the few tumours in which a virus can be seen to proliferate in the cell nucleus. The different types of wart caused by the many different types of papilloma viruses cannot be discussed here but certain aspects should be remembered.

(1) Genital warts (due to human papilloma virus) very rarely undergo malignant change but the associated infection of the cervix frequently leads to dysplasia or malignant changes. Cervical smears must be taken.

(2) Very extensive proliferation of warts occurs in patients receiving immunosuppressive therapy, such as renal transplant recipients, and in patients with AIDS.

(3) Epidermodysplasia verruciformis, an unusual widespread eruption of erythematous warty plaques, can develop into carcinoma.

Treatment

Most warts occur in childen and resolve spontaneously without treatment or with very simple measures. These include paints or lotions containing salicylic and lactic acids and formalin in various proportions, which should be applied daily. Salicylic acid (40%) plasters are useful for plantar warts; they are cut to shape and held in place with sticking plaster for two or three days. Glutaraldehyde solution is also used.

For warts that get in the way, are painful, or are disfiguring more drastic measures can be used.

(1) *Cold*—Carbon dioxide snow is readily produced from a cylinder and can be mixed with acetone to form a slush. This is applied with a cotton wool swab. Liquid nitrogen is colder and more effective but has to be stored in special containers and replaced frequently. It can be applied with cotton wool or discharged from a special spray apparatus. Freezing is continued until there is a rim of frozen tissue around the wart but not for more than 30 seconds. Subsequent blistering may occur. Scarring is unusual.

Treatment.

(2) *Heat*—Cautery causes more scarring and requires local anaesthesia. The diathermy loop is effective for perianal warts.

(3) *Curettage and cautery* together are effective but leave scars and the warts may recur.

(4) *Podophyllin*, 15%–25% in tincture of benzoin compound or alcoholic solution, is effective for genital warts when applied each week. It is, however, toxic when ingested or absorbed and must never be used in pregnancy.

Other treatments include radiotherapy, fluorouracil, and bleomycin injections. Hypnosis has been effectively used, and fear of painful treatment has caused warts to fall off.

Virus diseases with rashes

    Measles
    Rubella
    Infectious mononucleosis
    Erythema infectiosum
    Roseola infantum
    Gianotti-Crosti syndrome
    Hand, foot, and mouth disease
    Primary HIV infection

Measles and rubella, which were once familiar to every doctor, are now much less common as a result of widespread inoculation. However, measles is probably the best known example of an exanthem (a fever characterised by a skin eruption. In an enanthem the mucous surfaces are affected). Other common clinical patterns can then be compared with it. All exanthems, except fifth disease (erythema infectiosum), are due to RNA viruses.

Measles

Age—Measles affects children, usually those aged over 5.

Incubation lasts seven to 14 days.

Prodromal symptoms include fever, malaise, upper respiratory symptoms; conjunctivitis; and photophobia.

Initial rash—Early on Koplik's spots (white spots with surrounding erythema) appear on the oral mucosa. After two days a macular rash appears on the face, trunk, and limbs. Look behind the ears for early lesions.

Development and resolution—The rash becomes papular, with coalescence. There may be haemorrhagic lesions and bullae which fade to leave brown patches.

Complications are encephalitis, otitis media, and bronchopneumonia.

Diagnosis—Specific antibodies may be detected; they are at their maximum at two to four weeks.

Rubella

Age—Rubella affects children and young adults.

Incubation lasts 14 to 21 days.

Prodromal symptoms—There are none in young children. Otherwise fever, malaise, and upper respiratory symptoms occur.

Initial rash—Initially some patients develop erythema of the soft palate and lymphadenopathy. Later pink macules appear on the face, spreading to trunk and limbs over one to two days.

Development and resolution—The rash then clears over the next two days, and sometimes no rash develops at all.

Complications—The main complication is congenital defects in babies of women infected during pregnancy. The risk is greatest in the first month.

Diagnosis—The diagnosis is made from the clinical signs above. Serum should be taken for measuring antibodies and the test repeated at seven to 10 days.

Prophylaxis—Active immunisation is now routinely available for all schoolgirls.

Erythema infectiosum (fifth disease)

Age group—Erythema infectiosum affects children aged 2–10 years, mainly girls.

Incubation lasts five to 20 days.

Prodromal symptoms—There are usually none, but there may be a slight fever with initial rash.

Initial rash—The initial rash is a hot, erythematous eruption on the cheeks—hence the "slapped cheek syndrome." Over two to four days a maculopapular eruption develops on the arms, legs, and trunk.

Development and resolution—The rash extends to affect hands, feet, and mucous membranes, then fades over one to two weeks.

Diagnosis is made by finding a specific IgM antibody to parvovirus B19.

Complications—There are no reported dermatological complications but haematological disorders, arthropathy, and fetal abnormalities may be associated.

Roseola infantum

Age group—Roseola infantum affects infants aged under 2.

Incubation lasts 10–15 days.

Prodromal symptoms—There is fever for a few days.

Initial rash—A rose pink maculopapular eruption appears on the neck and trunk.

Measles (left); rubella (below); Gianotti-Crosti syndrome (below left); hand, foot, and mouth disease (below right).

Development and resolution—The rash may affect the face and limbs before clearing over one to two days.

Diagnosis—The condition is diagnosed from its clinical features.

Complications include febrile convulsions.

Gianotti-Crosti syndrome

Age group—The Gianotti-Crosti syndrome affects children, usually those aged under 14.

Incubation period is unknown.

Prodromal symptoms—Lymphadenopathy and malaise accompany the eruption.

Initial rash—Red papules rapidly develop on the face, neck, limbs, buttocks, palms, and soles.

Development and resolution—Over two to three weeks the lesions become purpuric then slowly fade.

Diagnosis—The syndrome may be due to a number of virus infections. Check for hepatitis B antigen.

Complications—Lymphadenopathy and hepatomegaly always occur and may persist for many months.

Hand, foot, and mouth disease

Age—Hand, foot, and mouth disease (Coxsackie virus A) affects both children and adults.

Incubation period is unknown.

Prodromal symptoms—Fever, headache, and malaise may accompany the rash.

Initial rash—Initially there may be intense erythema surrounding yellow-grey vesicles; ulceration then occurs. This pattern is more common in adults. Alternatively, there may be grey vesicles, 1–5 mm diameter, with surrounding erythema on the palms and soles. These occur mainly in children, in whom a more generalised eruption may develop.

Development and resolution—Over three to five days the rash fades.

Diagnosis—Coxsackie A (usually A16) virus is isolated from lesions and stools. A specific antibody may be found in the serum.

Complications are rare but include widespread vesicular rashes and erythema multiforme.

Other infections

Secondary syphilis.

Infectious mononucleosis—As well as the erythematous lesions on the palate a maculopapular rash affecting the face and limbs can occur.

Cat scratch disease—A crusted nodule at the site of the scratch is associated with development of regional lymphadenopathy one or two months later. A maculopapular eruption on the face and limbs or erythema multiforme may occur.

Psittacosis and ornithosis may be associated with a rash.

Rickettsial infections, including typhus, Rocky Mountain spotted fever, and Rickettsial pox are all associated with rashes.

Syphilis—Although not a viral infection, the transient roseolar rash of secondary syphilis is followed by a papulosquamous eruption, which affects the trunk, limbs, and mucous membranes. The palms and soles may be affected. The diagnosis should always be considered in any rash that does not fit a recognised pattern.

HIV and AIDS

Seborrhoeic dermatitis.

Herpes zoster with oral candidiasis.

Oral hairy leukoplakia.

Since AIDS was first described in 1981 over 400 000 cases have been reported to the World Health Organisation, but the total is probably much larger. In Europe the figure is over 60 000, of which 5000 are from the United Kingdom. The number of people infected with HIV is much larger. It is generally accepted that this retrovirus is the causative agent of AIDS, but its origins remain unknown.

Skin lesions occur in patients with AIDS:
(1) As a manifestaton of the primary HIV infection.
(2) As a consequence of immunosuppression (AIDS).

Between these two events there is a latent period that can last from a few months to several years. Lymphadenopathy may occur without other signs of the disease.

Acute HIV infection (seroconversion illness) is associated with clinical changes in about a half of cases. Fever, malaise, headache, lymphadenopathy, and gastrointestinal upset occur. Sometimes there is an effect on the central nervous system. Soon after the onset of these effects a transient maculopapular eruption occurs, with erythema and erosion of the palate in some patients. At this time HIV can be isolated from circulating lymphocytes and HIV antibody testing may still give negative results, although an antigenaemia soon develops. For this reason it may be important to retest suspected cases 6–8 weeks later. Counselling should take place when testing is carried out.

Skin manifestations of AIDS and late stage HIV disease are many and variable. The main features are that the common inflammatory skin diseases are more florid, infections are frequent and severe, and opportunistic infections occur. In addition Kaposi's sarcoma occurs in 34% of homosexual men and in 5% of other cases.

Seborrhoeic eczema is common and may be the only evidence of HIV infection initially. It is more extensive and inflamed than usual. The role of *Pityrosporum* organisms is indicated by the response to imidazole antifungal drugs.

Psoriasis is more widespread, severe, and resistant to treatment in patients with late HIV disease. The use of ultraviolet light may lead to an increased risk of Kaposi's sarcoma.

Any type of opportunistic infection is more likely in patients with AIDS and will generally be more severe.

An itching, *inflammatory folliculitis* occurs in many cases. The cause is unknown, but it is possible that *Demodex* spp play a part.

Herpes zoster virus infection is common, with florid lesions and systemic spread. Often two dermatomes are affected. *Herpes simplex virus* produces widespread and sometimes persistent ulcerating lesions.

Perianal warts can proliferate and *cervical intraepithelial neoplasia* occurs. *Molluscum contagiosum* is often widespread, particularly on the face.

HIV and AIDS

Kaposi's sarcoma.

Kaposi's sarcoma of the hard palate.

Fungal infections may be widespread and with increased inflammation and hyperkeratosis. *Candidiasis*, often with associated bacterial infection, is very common, particularly at the corners of the mouth, on the palate, and in the pharynx.

Cryptococcus neoformans and *Histoplasma capsulatum* are occasional opportunistic pathogens and can produce inflammatory, papular, and necrotic lesions.

Mycobacteria may cause both cutaneous and systemic lesions.

Oral hairy leukoplakia may occur in 30%–50% of patients with AIDS.

Kaposi's sarcoma presents with polychromic plaques and nodules, varying from red and purple to brown. They are common on the palate and nose, often found on the trunk, but can be disseminated or produce lesions in the classical site—the ankle.

AIDS may thus present with a wide variety of skin conditions, commonly with several present at the same time. Any unusually florid skin condition that is resistant to treatment should raise the suspicion that HIV infection may be present.

FUNGAL AND YEAST INFECTIONS

Fungal infections

Trubrum infection of the neck.

Animal ringworm.

Tinea cruris.

T mentagrophytes.

M canis.

Fungal infection of nail.

Fungal infections are commonly known as "ringworm"—a misnomer since most infections cause a scaling macule, not a ring, and the worm exists only in the imagination. It is true, however, that a superficial fungal infection can have a raised edge, and annular forms occur.

Fungi consist of thread-like hyphae—which form tangled masses, or mycelia, in the common moulds. In "dermatophyte" fungal infection of the skin, hair, and nails these hyphae invade keratin and are seen on microscopic examination of keratin from infected tissues. Vegetative spores (conidia) develop in culture, and their distinctive shape helps to differentiate one species from another.

Systemic, or deep, fungal infection is due to those species that invade other tissues. When the immune response is impaired superficial infections may invade the deeper tissues.

Yeasts are budding unicellular organisms that do not normally produce hyphae. The commonest infective species in humans is *Candida albicans*.

Why should one suspect a lesion to be due to a fungus?

Clinical presentation

Fungal infections usually itch. Those due to zoophilic (animal) fungi produce a more intense inflammatory response with deeper indurated lesions than those due to anthropophilic (human) species. In those lesions with a raised scaling margin that extends outwards the fungal hyphae are invading the keratin layer in this area. The central area is relatively resistant to colonisation. Such lesions occur mainly on the trunk.

Children below the age of puberty rarely develop anthropophilic (human) fungal infection. In the countryside cattle ringworm (zoophilic) infects children in the autumn when the cows are brought into winter quarters. Pet mice can also be a source of infection.

Adults—From adolescence onwards infection of the feet, not only in athletes, occurs. Tinea cruris in the groin is seen mainly in men.

Infection from cattle occurs in adults who have not had previous exposure, sometimes in unusual ways. A man who lived in an industrial area housing estate developed a curious indurated lesion on his chin from which *Trichophyton mentagrophytes* was isolated—transmitted by bites from midges who had been biting cows on a farm some miles away.

Infection from dogs and cats with a zoophilic fungus (*Microsporum canis*) to which humans have little immunity can occur at any age. A colleague's daughter returned from a skiing holiday with intensely itchy "eczema," which refused to clear. A stray kitten, mewing outside in the dark, had been taken indoors, warmed in their sleeping bags, and infected the whole party with *M canis*.

Nail infections occur mainly in adults, usually in their toenails, especially when traumatised—for example, the big toes of footballers. The nails become thickened and yellow and crumble, usually asymmetrically. The changes occur *distally* and move back to the nailfold. In psoriasis of the nail the changes occur *proximally* and tend to be symmetrical and are associated with pitting and other evidence of psoriasis elsewhere.

Chronic paronychia occurs in the fingers of individuals whose work demands repeated wetting of the hands: housewives, barmen, dentists, nurses, and mushroom growers, for example. Other predisposing

Fungal and yeast infections

Chronic paronychia.

factors include diabetes, poor peripheral circulation, and removal of the cuticle. There is erythema and swelling of the nail fold, often on one side with brownish discoloration of the nail. Pus may be exuded. The cause is *Candida albicans* (a yeast) together with secondary bacterial infection.

Pushing back the cuticles should be avoided. It is commonly a long term condition, lasting for years. The hands should be kept as dry as possible, nystatin cream applied regularly, and, if necessary a course of erythromycin prescribed.

Tinea pedis.

Feet—It is not only athletes and the unhygienic who suffer from athletes' foot but increased sweating does predispose to infection. The hands may be affected, often through scratching the feet; hence the "right hand, left foot" syndrome in the right handed individual. The itching, macerated skin beneath the toes is familiar, but when a dry, scaling rash extends across the sole and dorsal surface of one foot the diagnosis may be missed. The condition needs to be differentiated from psoriasis and eczema.

Hands—Fungal infections often produce a dry, hot, rash on one palm. There may be well defined lesions with a scaling edge.

Tinea corporis.　　　Erythrasma.

Trunk—Tinea corporis presents with erythema and itching and a well defined scaling edge. The infection may spread to the adjacent skin on the thighs and abdomen. Intense erythema and satellite lesions suggest a candida infection. In the axillae erythrasma due to *Corynebacterium minutissimum* is more likely. It does not respond to antifungal treatment but clears with tetracycline by mouth.

M audouini.

Scalp and face—The classic scalp ringworm of children due to *Microsporum audouini* is rare. Favus, a scarring type of alopecia, caused by *Trichophyton schoenleini*, and "black dot" ringworm, also from a trichophyton, are now seen only in children who have acquired the infection abroad. In all cases there is itching, hair loss, and some degree of inflammation. *M. canis* from dogs and cats can affect the scalp.

Kerion—an inflamed, boggy, pustular lesion, is due to cattle ringworm and is fairly common in rural areas. It is often seen in children in the autumn when the cows are brought inside for the winter.

"Tinea incognito" is the term used for unrecognised fungal infection in patients treated with steroids (topical or systemic). The normal response to infection (leading to erythema, scaling, a raised margin, and itching) is diminished, particularly with local steroid creams or ointments. The infecting organism flourishes, however, because of the host's impaired immune response—shown by the enlarging, persistent skin lesions. The groins, hands, and face are sites where this is most likely to occur.

Deep fungal infection

Fungal infection of the deeper tissues is rare in the United Kingdom but is of course a feature of AIDS. The species that colonise the deep tissue, as in histoplasmosis, actinomycosis, and cryptococcosis, can also cause skin lesions. In any patient with chronic indurated inflammatory lesions the possibility of deep fungal infection should be considered.

Tinea incognito.　　　Actinomycosis.

Tinea versicolor.

Tinea versicolor affects the trunk, usually of fair skinned individuals exposed to the sun. It affects mainly the upper back, chest, and arms. Well defined macular lesions with fine scales develop which tend to be white in suntanned areas and brown on pale skin (hence "versicolor"—variable colour). It may be confused with seborrhoeic dermatitis, pityriasis rosea, and vitiligo.

In skin scrapings the causative organism, *Pityrosporum* spp—normally found in hair follicles—can be readily seen.

Yeast infections

Candida albicans.

Candida infection may occur in the flexures of infants and elderly or immobilised patients, especially below the breasts and folds of abdominal skin. It needs to be differentiated from (*a*) psoriasis, which does not itch; (*b*) seborrhoeic dermatitis, the usual cause of a flexural rash in infants; and (*c*) contact dermatitis and discoid eczema, which do not have the scaling margin. It is symmetrical.

Yeasts, including *Candida albicans*, may be found in the mouth and vagina of healthy individuals. Clinical lesions may be produced by local trauma predisposing factors including: general debilitation, impaired immunity, diabetes mellitus, endocrine disorders, particularly Cushing's syndrome, and corticosteroid treatment. Florid mucocutaneous lesions can occur in which mycelial forms of *Candida albicans* are found.

Principles of diagnosis and treatment

(1) Consider a fungal infection in any patient where isolated, itching, dry, and scaling lesions occur without any apparent reason—for example, if there is no previous history of eczema. Lesions due to fungal infection are often asymmetrical.

(2) Skin scrapings should be sent to the laboratory from any suspicious lesion and are easy to take. The skin scales should be removed by scraping the edge of the lesion with a scalpel at right angles to the skin on to a piece of folded black paper. A strip of Sellotape applied to the lesion then stuck on a slide gives the laboratory more material for culture. Some laboratories supply mycology kits containing black paper, a slide with Sellotape, and suitable plastic containers. Clippings can be taken from the nails.

(3) Lesions to which steroids have been applied are often quite atypical because the normal inflammatory response is suppressed—tinea incognito. The patient often states that the treatment controls the itch but the contagion lingers on, becoming worse when the steroid is stopped. This may also occur in eczema being treated with steroids.

(4) Wood's light (ultraviolet light filtered through special glass) can be used to show microsporum infections, which produce a green-blue fluorescence.

Treatment

Topical treatment—The old fashioned treatment with Whitfield's ointment (benzoic acid ointment, compound) is quite effective, but has been superseded by the new imidazole preparations, such as clotrimazole and miconazole and also by terbinafine. The polyenes, nystatin and amphotericin B are also effective against yeast infection. For damp macerated skin dusting powders or painting with Castellani's paint (magenta paint) is helpful. Terbinafine, a fungicidal drug, is available as a cream and is very effective.

Systemic treatment—Griseofulvin should be taken for an adequate length of time: three to four months for the trunk and scalp, six to eight months for finger nails, and at least a year for toenails, where it is often ineffective. It is important to confirm the diagnosis from scrapings before starting treatment. The dose is 500 mg daily for adults and 10 mg/kg for children (taken with food).

Contraindications to griseofulvin are pregnancy, liver failure, and porphyria. It interacts with the coumarin anticoagulants, and its effect is diminished with barbiturates. Imidazole preparations such as ketoconazole are effective in both dermatophyte fungi and yeast infections. Cases of liver damage have, however, been reported. Fluconazole is effective in yeast infections. Some drugs interact with azole drugs, the main ones being anticoagulants, oral hypoglycaemic drugs, phenytoin, and theophylline. Terbinafine is a new antifungal drug that is safe and a very effective fungicidal drug. It will probably become the treatment of choice.

INSECT BITES AND INFESTATIONS

Body louse.

Leishmaniasis.

It is, of course, the internal parasites of biting insects that cause trouble for humans, rather than "smaller fleas" on their surface.

An ornithologist went bird watching in Guyana, where he sustained widespread "midge bites" on the arms. He was referred on account of nodules that developed a few weeks later, then enlarged and ulcerated. Other lesions occurred further up the arms with regional lymphadenopathy. A biopsy specimen showed histiocytic inflammatory changes, and *Leishmania braziliensis* was isolated from smears; the midges (*phlebotomus* or sand fly) had acquired the protozoon while feeding on local rodents and transferred it into the ornithologist's skin.

Serious disease from insect vectors is rare in residents of most Western countries but, as in the patient described above, must be considered in those returning from tropical and subtropical countries.

Most cases of bites from fleas, midges, and mosquitoes are readily recognised and cause few symptoms apart from discomfort. Occasionally an allergic reaction confuses the picture, particularly the large bullae that can occur from bites on the arms and legs. It may be difficult to persuade patients that their recurrent itching spots are simply due to flea bites and the suggestion may be angrily rejected.

Some diseases with skin lesions resulting from insect bites

Condition	Appearance	Organism	Vector
Cutaneous leishmaniasis	Chronic enlarging nodules with ulceration	Leishmania protozoon (L braziliensis)	Sand fly
Oriental sore	Ulcerating nodules	Leishmania (L tropica)	Sand fly
Kala-azar	Hypopigmented, erythematous, and nodular lesions	Leishmania (L donovani)	Insect vectors
Onchocerciasis	Pruritic nodules	Filaria (Onchocerca volvulus)	Black fly (Simuliidae)
Typhus, human	Erythematous rash and systemic illness	Rickettsia (R prowazekii)	Human louse
Typhus, murine		(R mooseri)	Rat flea
Rocky Mountain spotted fever	Maculopapular rash and fever	Rickettsia (R rickettsii)	Ticks
Rickettsial pox	Vesicular eruption like chickenpox	Rickettsia (R akari)	House mouse, louse
Tick typhus	Necrotic lesions, maculopapular rash, and fever	Various rickettsias	Ticks
Scrub typhus	Fever, lymphadenopathy, maculopapular rash	Rickettsia (R tsutsugamushi)	Mites
Relapsing fever	Widespread maculopapular lesions	Borrelia recurrentis	Lice, ticks
Lyme disease	May be annular	Borrelia Burgdorferi	Ticks, black fly
Yellow fever and dengue	Flushing of face, scarlatiniform rash	Arbovirus	Aedes mosquito

Bullae caused by insect bites.

On the other hand, some patients are convinced that they have an infestation when they do not. Often they will bring small packets containing "insects." Examination shows these to be small screws of wool,

Parasitophobia specimens.

pickings of keratin, thread, and so on. Sympathy and tact will win patients' confidence; derision and disbelief will merely send them elsewhere for a further medical opinion. Pimozide by mouth may help to dispel the delusion of parasitic infestation (delusional parasitosis).

Some useful points:

(1) Flea bites, including those from *Cheyletiella* mites in dogs and cats, occur in clusters, often in areas of close contact with clothing—for example, around the waist.

(2) Grain mites (*Pyemotes*) and harvest mites (*Trombicula*) can cause severe reactions.

(3) Tick, and possibly mosquito, bites can produce infection with *Borrelia Burgdorferi*, causing arthropathy, fever, and a distinctive rash (erythema chronicum migrans)—Lyme disease. The condition responds rapidly to treatment with penicillin. Increasing numbers of cases are being reported in the United Kingdom.

Bites on ankles.

Erythema chronicum migrans.

Harvest mites.

Papular urticaria.

Persistent papules in scabies.

Papular urticaria

Persistent pruritic (itching) papules in groups on the trunk and legs may be due to bites from fleas, bed bugs, or mites. A seasonal incidence suggests bites from outdoor insects, while recurrence of the papules in a particular house or room suggests infestations with fleas. The term is sometimes used for other causes of itchy skin.

Spider bites

Spider bite (Nigeria).

In Europe spider bites rarely cause problems, but sometimes noxious species arrive in consignmnets of tropical fruit. The patient shown had been bitten by a spider the day before leaving Nigeria and developed a painful necrotic lesion.

Bites from the European tarantula are painful but otherwise harmless.

In tropical and subtropical countries venomous spiders inject neurotoxins that can be fatal. The "black widow" (*Latrodectus mactans*), "fiddleback" (*Loxosceles veclusa*), and *Atrax* species of Australia are better known examples. Scorpions cause severe local and systemic symptoms as a result of stings (not bites).

Infestations

Burrows of scabies.

Scabies

The commonest infestation encountered is scabies, and it is easily missed or misdiagnosed. Scabies is due to a small mite, *Sarcoptes scabiei*. The female mite burrows into the stratum corneum to lay her eggs; the male dies after completing his role of fertilisation, and the developing eggs hatch into larvae within a few days. Intense itching occurs some two weeks later, during which time extensive colonisation may have occurred. The infestation is acquired only by close contact with infected people.

Diagnosis—Finding a burrow—the small (5–10 mm long) ridge, often S shaped—can be difficult as it is often obscured by excoriation from scratching. Without finding a burrow, however, the diagnosis remains uncertain. Isolation of an acarus with a needle or scalpel blade and its demonstration under the microscope convinces the most sceptical patient. Always ask whether there are others in the patient's household and if any of them are itching.

Insect bits and infestations

Larva migrans.

Pediculosis capitis.

Head lice and nits.

Treatment—10% Sulphur in yellow soft paraffin is traditional, effective, and safe. There are several more modern treatments, including 25% benzyl benzoate emulsion, 0.5% malathion cream, 1% gamma benzene hexachloride (lindane) lotion, and 1% permethrin. In children benzyl benzoate should be diluted to 10% and used with care as toxicity results from absortion. In infants over 2 months old permethrin or 2.5% sulphur ointment can be used. Gamma benzene hexachloride should not be given to children under 10 or pregnant women in the first trimester. Important points are:

(1) The patient should wash well: a hot bath was formerly advocated but it is now known that this may increase absorption through the skin.

(2) The lotion should be applied from the neck down, concentrating on affected areas and making sure that the axillae, wrists, ankles, and pubic areas are included. If there is any doubt about the thoroughness of application the process should be repeated in a few days.

(3) All contacts and members of the patient's household should be treated at the same time.

(4) Residual papules may persist for many weeks. Topical steroids can be used to relieve the itching.

(5) Secondary infection as a result of scratching may need to be treated.

Demodex

Demodex folliculorum is a small mite that inhabits the human hair follicle, the eggs being deposited in the sebaceous gland. It is found on the central area of the face, chest, and neck of adults. It may have a role in the pathogenesis of rosacea, in which it may be found in large numbers. It may be associated with a pustular eruption round the mouth and blepharitis.

Larva migrans

The boy in the illustration had been on holiday at a coastal town in Kenya and regularly played on a beach frequented by dogs. Two weeks after returning to Britain he started itching on the buttocks and subsequently his parents noticed a linear, raised area that progressed to form a semicircle—a condition known as larva migrans, due to the larvae of the hookworm of dogs and cats, *Ancyclostoma caninum*. The ova are shed in the faeces and in a warm moist environment hatch into larvae that invade "dead end" hosts. They do not develop any further, so systemic disease does not occur.

Treatment—is either by freezing the advancing end of the lesion with liquid nitrogen or by applying thiabendazole (10%) suspension. Similar lesions in patients returning from tropical countries raises the possibility of larva migrans from strongyloides infestation, myiasis from the larvae of flies, or gnathostomiasis.

Visceral larva migrans caused by *Toxocara canis* and *Ascaris lumbricoides* may produce a transient rash.

Pediculosis (lice)

Infestation with lice became less common in the postwar years, but the incidence has recently increased.

There are three areas of the body usually affected by two speices of wingless insects—*Pediculus humanus*, infecting the head and body, and *Phthirus pubis*, the pubic louse. The wingless insects feed on blood aspirated at the site of the bite, and each female lays 60–80 encapsulated eggs attached to hairs—"nits" in common parlance.

Head lice are transmitted via combs, brushes, and hats, being more common in girls than boys. The infestation is heaviest behind the ears and over the occiput. If the eyelashes of children are affected this is with "crab lice" (*Phthirus pubis*); it is not pediculosis.

Body lice are less common in western Europe. Transmission is by clothing and bedding, on which both lice and their eggs may be found in the seams. Poor hygiene favours infestation.

Pubic lice infestation occurs world wide and is generally transmitted by sexual contact. Infestation of eyelashes may occur with poor hygiene.

As a result of scratching there may be marked secondary infection that obscures the underlying infestation.

Treatment—Gamma benzene hexachloride 1% is usually effective as a single application. Permethrin can also be used.

DISEASES OF THE HAIR AND SCALP

D Kemmett

The growth cycle

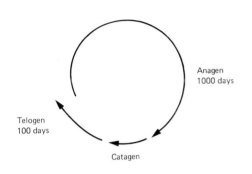

Telogen
100 days

Anagen
1000 days

Catagen

Hair has no vital function in humans, but the lack or excess of it may cause endless misery. Minor "faults" in hair texture, colour, or shape sustain an industry worth billions of pounds a year.

Each hair on the body goes through a cycle of growth independent of its neighbours. The length of each phase of the cycle, as well as its overall length, varies with site and age. For example, the scalp anagen, the growing phase, averages 1000 days; catagen, when the follicles involute, only a few days; and telogen, a resting state, 100 days. An average scalp contains 100 000 hairs and sheds about 100 "naturally" each day.

There are also long term trends in hair growth: the number of follicles decreases with age, having been maximal at birth.

Telogen effluvium is a common type of diffuse hair loss occurring after pregnancy or after a severe illness. During pregnancy, most hairs move into anagen. After delivery large numbers of these follicles involute (catagen phase) and pass into the resting state, in which no further growth occurs. When anagen starts again, some eight weeks later, the resting hairs are pushed out and lost, causing a temporary diffuse thinning of scalp hair.

Anagen effluvium follows any insult to the hair follicle which cuts down mitosis or weakens the hair shaft. This is the usual way in which drugs cause alopecia.

Hormonal factors—Hair follicles are under hormonal control: androgens and thyroxine are the most important hormones but many others influence them to some extent. All hair is sensitive to androgens, but this is most striking in the secondary sexual hair of the axillae, pubis, and face.

Diseases of the hair fall into three groups:
* Excess hair—hirsutism, hypertrichosis
* Hair loss—alopecia
* Deformity of hair shafts

Anagen effluvium.

Diffuse alopecia caused by cyclosporin.

Excess of hair

Causes of hirsutism	
• Hereditary, racial	
• Endocrine	
Adrenal	—virilising tumours Cushing's syndrome adrenal hyperplasia
Ovarian	—virilising tumours polycystic ovary syndrome
Pituitary	—acromegaly hyperprolactinaemia
• Iatrogenic	—anabolic steroids, androgens, corticosteroids, danazol, phenytoin, psoralens (in PUVA)

Hirsutism is an excess of coarse secondary sexual hair in a male distribution. *Hypertrichosis* is an excessive growth in any other pattern.

Idiopathic or hereditary causes are by far the most common causes of hirsutism, especially in women from Mediterranean or Arabic countries. The prevalence of hirsutism also increases with age, and even in Caucasians it is common over the age of 60. There is usually a family history and general health is normal. Endocrine investigation is not needed.

Endocrine disease as a cause of hirsutism is rare but should be considered if the hirsutism develops rapidly or if it is associated with obvious virilisation, menstrual disturbances, infertility, or acne. Measurements of serum testosterone and urinary 17-oxosteroid concentrations are useful screening tests.

Treatment—The treatment of idiopathic hirsutism includes:
(*a*) depilatory creams or shaving; there is no evidence that these lead to increased growth or pigmentation of the hair;
(*b*) electrolysis and diathermy;
(*c*) in severe cases, the antiandrogen cyproterone, but this should be used only under specialist supervision.

Excess hair in men is seldom a problem.

Causes of hypertrichosis

- Congenital (rare)
- Acquired—porphyria
    hyperthyroidism
    anorexia nervosa
    some developmental defects
        eg Hurler's syndrome
    tumours (hypertrichosis
        lanuginosa)
    drugs (diazoxide, minoxidil,
        cyclosporin)

Hypertrichosis is rare and usually has an obvious cause. Treatment is directed to any underlying problem.

Hirsuties due to virilising tumour.

Hypertrichosis caused by minoxidil.

Alopecia

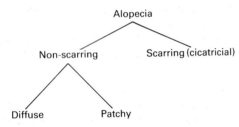

Alopecia can be classified into scarring or non-scarring types and the non-scarring types into diffuse or patchy. Scarring alopecia is usually associated with a concurrent skin disease, whereas in non-scarring alopecia the primary process affects the hair follicle.

Destruction of the hair follicle leads to plugging, atrophy (a fine and wrinkled appearance), and loss of the normally visible follicular orifices. The microscopic examination of plucked hairs may be useful, as may be a skin biopsy.

Remember that alopecia may reflect an underlying systemic disease or be a local manifestation of a generalised skin disease. A full history and examination are essential.

Causes of diffuse non-scarring alopecia

- Androgenetic
    alopecia—male pattern
        —female pattern
- Endocrine—thyroid disease
        (hypothyroidism and
        hyperthyroidism)
    —hypopituitarism
    —diabetes mellitus
- Stress —postpartum
    —postoperative } telogen effluvium
    —postfebrile
- Drugs —cytotoxics
    —anticoagulants
    —antithyroid } anagen effluvium
        agents
    —cyclosporin
- Erythrodermic skin
    disease —psoriasis
        —eczema
        —lymphoma
- Deficiency
    states —protein malnutrition
        —iron deficiency

Non-scarring alopecia

Androgenetic alopecia (common baldness) in men starts with frontotemporal thinning and then loss from the crown. These bald areas gradually become confluent, leaving only a rim of hair round the edge of the scalp. In women the pattern is more often diffuse and starts later and only rarely does the pattern resemble that of men. Testosterone is responsible but measuring serum concentrations is unhelpful because the underlying cause is hypersensitivity of the hair follicles to normal circulating concentrations of the hormone.

Men   Women

Treatment is ineffective. The value of topical minoxidil is limited. Meanwhile the "virility" theory (in men) may help some.

In hypothyroidism the hair is coarse, dry, and thin. Often the first indication is that the hair does not take a perm as it should.

Telogen and anagen effluvium have been discussed earlier.

Male pattern baldness.

Diffuse alopecia caused by erythrodermic psoriasis.

Causes of non-scarring alopecia

- Alopecia areata
- Trauma—trichotillomania
- Traction—hair straighteners, rollers
- Severe tinea infection

Patchy alopecia

Alopecia areata accounts for 2% of dermatological referrals in the United Kingdom. The peak incidence is in early adulthood. It is associated with autoimmune disease and with atopy. There is evidence of an immunological attack on the hair follicle.

There are usually no other signs apart from the alopecia and, sometimes, a slight erythema. The typical exclamation mark hairs are helpful in diagnosis.

Alopecia totalis.

Alopecia areata, showing exclamation mark hairs.

Alopecia areata.

The prognosis is unpredictable; often the hairs regrow after a few weeks. However, a gradual loss of scalp hair may lead to total alopecia. In severe cases the body hair may also be lost. Rapid evolution, loss of hair from the eyebrows, alopecia totalis, or loss of occipital hair are poor prognostic factors.

Treatment is disappointing. The injection of intralesional triamcinolone may induce a temporary regrowth and help psychologically. Permanent regrowth may not be achieved.

Trichotillomania.

Traction alopecia.

Trichotillomania is the constant plucking of hair by a patient who may be psychologically disturbed. The unusual pattern and the mental state of the patient usually makes the diagnosis straightforward. Treatment is often unsuccessful.

Traction alopecia is caused by an abnormal tug on the hair shafts from hairdressing accessories, such as tight rollers.

Scarring (cicatricial) alopecia

Hair follicles can be destroyed in several ways (see box). Acute inflammation is usually of infective origin. In preantibiotic days the moth eaten alopecia of syphilis was common.

Lupus erythematosus may affect the scalp in both its discoid and systemic forms. In the discoid type a heavy scale is seen with plugging of the hair follicles. A similar picture occurs in lichen planus, and the rash of lichen planus may be seen more typically elsewhere. Morphoea (localised scleroderma) may affect the scalp, the *en coup de sabre* pattern being one variant.

Causes of scarring alopecia

- Trauma —eg burns
- Inflammation
  Acute —bacterial (pyogenic infection, syphilis)
  —viral (herpes simplex, herpes zoster, varicella)
  —fungal (kerion caused by animal ringworm)
  Chronic —lupus erythematosus,
  —lichen planus
  —morphoea
  Rare —pyoderma gangrenosum
  —necrobiosis lipoidica
  —sarcoidosis

Systemic lupus erythematosus.

En coup de sabre.

A slowly extending area of alopecia may suggest a cicatricial basal cell carcinoma.

The treatment of scarring alopecia must be swift and directed at its underlying cause. Once scarring is present alopecia is irreversible. Potent topical steroids help in lupus erythematosus and lichen planus.

Hair shaft defects

Monilethrix.

Defects of the hair shaft are rare disorders leading to weakness or breaking of the hairs. Often they are inherited. The hairs may have a distinctive appearance, most evident on microscopy.

Examples of these defects include monilethrix and pili torti. Treatment is unsatisfactory.

Diseases of the scalp

The scalp is the site of predilection for several skin diseases, which are listed in the box, but seldom is the scalp the only site affected. Some have been dealt with under scarring alopecia and others in previous chapters.

Pityriasis capitis is the commonest skin complaint after acne, and indeed a mild dandruff is physiological. Reactions to *Pityrosporum ovale*, a normal yeast commensal, may play a part in its pathogenesis. Occasionally masses of sticky scale may heap up, matting adjacent hairs together. This picture is known as *pityriasis amiantacea*. A similar appearance may be seen in scalp psoriasis. The treatment of pityriasis capitis includes tar and salicylic acid preparations, and shampoos containing selenium, zinc pyrithione, or ketoconazole.

Diseases of the scalp

- *Infection and infestation*
  Bacterial—staphylococci, streptococci
  Viral—herpes zoster, herpes simplex, warts, molluscum
  Fungal—dermatophyte
  Pediculosis

- *Other conditions*
  Eczema—atopic dermatitis
  —seborrhoeic dermatitis, pityriasis capitis
  —contact dermatitis (hair dyes, formaldehyde)
  —neurodermatitis

  Psoriasis
  Other skin diseases—lupus erythematosus
  —lichen planus
  —morphoea
  Bullous diseases—pemphigoid
  —pemphigus
  —dermatitis herpetiformis
  Neoplasms, naevi, and cysts

Left: tinea capitis; right: pityriasis amiantacea.

Atopic eczema.   Contact eczema, hair dye.

DISEASES OF THE NAILS

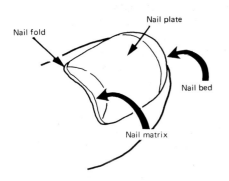

Nail fold — Nail plate — Nail bed — Nail matrix

A L Wright

Nails are a protective cover for the ends of the fingers and toes which also help increase tactile sensitivity by exerting counterpressure over the distal pulp.

The nail consists of a nail plate resting on the nail bed, which grows out from a nail matrix.

Fingernails grow about 1 cm in three months and toenails at about a third of this rate. Growth is slower in the non-dominant hand and in old age.

Examination and surface changes

Pits

Psoriasis
Alopecia
Hand dermatitis

Horizontal ridging

Beau's lines
Previous systemic illness
Hand dermatitis

> *Longitudinal ridges*
>
> *Single*
> Pressure effect
> *Multiple*
> Lichen planus
> Alopecia areata
> Psoriasis
> Darier's disease

A thorough relevant history is essential. Particular attention should be paid to past skin conditions because a previous episode of hand dermatitis may have settled leaving perplexing nail changes. A family history of psoriasis may explain nail changes in the absence of any other such signs. Occupation may also be relevant.

The nails should always be examined in adequate light, and all the fingernails and toenails should be inspected. Particular attention should be paid to the symmetry of the changes. For example, onychomycosis and psoriasis may cause similar changes, but psoriasis is commonly symmetrical while onychomycosis is often not.

Other signs of skin disease should be carefully looked for. Psoriasis can cause severe nail changes with no other skin lesions, but a thorough examination may show a small patch of psoriasis on the trunk or in the perianal area.

An assessment should then be made of which parts of the nail are affected. Are the changes in the surface texture of the nail, the nail plate itself, the nail bed, or the surrounding soft tissues?

Pits are small punctate depressions in the nail plate. They vary considerably in size and may be regular or irregular. They occur commonly in psoriasis, usually irregularly distributed, and in alopecia areata, when they may be very regular. They are less commonly associated with hand dermatitis.

Horizontal ridging is usually seen in the form of Beau's line. This is usually a single horizontal depression that progresses distally with nail growth and indicates a previous episode of illness. Multiple small horizontal ridges may occur with hand dermatitis or any inflammatory condition affecting the soft tissues around the nail.

Longitudinal ridges—Single longitudinal ridges may be caused by pressure from tumours, either benign or malignant, in the proximal nail fold. These may progress to a true split in the nail.

Diseases of the nails

Trachyonychia

Lichen planus
Psoriasis
Alopecia areata

Multiple longitudinal ridges of varying size are a feature of lichen planus, psoriasis, alopecia areata, and Darier's disease. When lichen planus is suspected the buccal mucosal membrane should always be examined for lesions.

Trachyonychia is roughness of the nails, so that they feel like fine sandpaper. This change is usually symmetrical and can occur in lichen planus, psoriasis, and alopecia areata.

Changes in the nail plate

Thickening

Psoriasis
Onychomycosis
Pachyonychia congenita

Lamellar splitting
Trauma

Shedding—onychomadesis

Systemic illness
Lichen planus

Thickening or hypertrophy of the nail plate is most commonly seen with psoriasis and onychomycosis. The changes are often asymmetrical. The presence of other nail changes due to psoriasis (such as pitting and onycholysis) should be sought if there are no other skin signs of psoriasis. Nail clippings may need to be taken for microscopy and culture to exclude fungal infection. More rarely the changes may affect all the nails as in pachyonychia congenita.

Lamellar splitting of the nail plate occurs distally and horizontally and is caused by exogenous factors, particularly repeated immersion in water.

Onychomadesis is complete shedding of the nail and can occur in any severe illness which results in sudden stopping of nail growth. The nail plate continues to move distally and is shed when it loses its adhesion to underlying tissues. This change may rarely occur with lichen planus. Shedding may be seen with any condition which causes severe onycholysis.

Detachment—onycholysis

Psoriasis
Onychomycosis
Trauma
Thyrotoxicosis

Thickening—onychogryphosis

Trauma

Subungual hyperkeratosis

Psoriasis
Hand dermatitis

Onycholysis is detachment of the nail from its bed. The main difference from onychomadesis is that it usually, but not always, begins distally or laterally, causing a subungual space which fills with air, giving that area of the nail a whitish grey discoloration. It is most commonly seen in psoriasis but can occur in onychomycosis, thyrotoxicosis, and trauma. It may become extensive, enough to cause nail loss, through loosening of the nail plate.

Onychogryphosis is thickening of the nail, probably due to repeated trauma. It commonly affects the nails of both great toes but may affect other toes as well.

Subungual hyperkeratosis is due to hyperplasia of the epidermis underlying the nail plate and occurs either distally or throughout the nail. It is usually seen in psoriasis and hand dermatitis.

Colour changes in the nail plate—Apparent changes in colour may be caused by changes in the nail bed. Cyanosis may make the nails look blue. Actual discoloration of the nail plate can be due to endogenous or exogenous factors. *Exogenous* factors include occupational exposure to dyes or other materials. Infection with pseudomonas may colour the nail green and topical treatment may stain the nail plate—for example, potassium permanganate soaks stain it brown. Prolonged application of nail varnish may also make nails brown. *Endogenous* causes of discoloration include a wide variety of drugs and systemic illnesses.

Leukonychia

True
Onychomycosis
Trauma

Apparent
Anaemia
Hypoproteinaemia

Colour changes

Exogenous
Occupational
Pseudomonas infection
Topical treatment

Endogenous
Drugs, eg
  Tetracyclines—yellow
  Antimalarials—blue
  Chlorpromazine—
    brown
Systemic illness, eg
  Jaundice—yellow
  Cirrhosis—white
  Adrenal
    insufficiency—
    brown

Koilonychia

Iron deficiency

Pigmented streaks

Malignant melanoma

**Normal in pigmented
  skin**
Melanocytic naevi
Lentigo
Addison's disease

Koilonychia is a spoon shaped deformity of the nail plate, which may also be thinned. The changes may be asymmetrical. The fingers are usually more affected than the toes. It is most characteristically seen in association with iron deficiency anaemia but may be idiopathic.

Leukonychia or whiteness of the nails is said to be true when it affects the nail plate and apparent when it affects the subungual tissues. Complete whiteness of the nail is rare, but isolated total leukonychia is seen with fungal infections. The only common form of true leukonychia is the punctate form, which occurs as small white spots 1–3 mm in diameter, singly or in groups. This probably relates to episodes of trauma to the nail matrix. Apparent leukonychia is seen in anaemia and hypoproteinaemia.

Pigmented streaks—Longitudinal pigmented streaks may be multiple in pigmented skin and are a normal finding. Their presence in white people, particularly if of recent onset, raises the possibility of a malignant melanoma of the nail. These may or may not produce dystrophic changes in the nail plate. Twenty five per cent of subungual melanomas are amelanotic. Other causes of pigmented streaks include conditions such as a lentigo, as well as benign melanocytic naevi. Similar changes may be seen in Addison's disease.

Around the nail: soft tissue changes

Paronychia

Acute
Trauma

Chronic
Trauma
Water

Pterygium formation

Circulatory disorders
Lichen planus

Paronychia is probably the commonest of nail complaints. When it occurs acutely it usually begins at the side of the nail with redness and swelling. Pus may collect which requires drainage. The commonest infecting organisms are staphylococci and less commonly β haemolytic streptococci. Correct antibiotic therapy is essential.

The condition may present as a more chronic problem characterised by loss of the cuticle over all or part of the nail with thickening of the nail fold and variable inflammation.

Acute paronychia usually affects only one nail, whereas chronic paronychias may affect several. The cause may also be different. Acute paronychia is often related to minor trauma whereas the chronic state usually results from repeated immersion in water, and *Candida albicans* can be isolated in many cases, together with Gram positive cocci and Gram negative bacteria.

Pterygium formation—The cuticle appears to grow out over the nail with loss of the proximal nail fold. Initially this may appear to split the nail but can progress to complete nail loss. It is due to a scarring loss of the nail matrix and is seen in conditions characterised by impairment of the circulation and occasionally in lichen planus.

Treatment of nail disorders

> ### Treatment of chronic paronychia
> - Keep hands as dry as possible
> - Treat episodes of inflammation with oral antibiotics
> - Long term application of ointment containing nystatin or antiseptic paint, eg gentian violet

Fungal infection.

Further reading

Samman PD, Fenton DA. *The nails in disease.* 4th ed. London: Heinemann, 1986.

Baran R, Barth J, Dawber RPR. *Nail disorders: common presenting signs, differential diagnosis and treatment.* London: Dunitz, 1990.

Few specific treatments are successful for nail disorders, except for fungal infections. First line treatment is still probably with griseofulvin. This may need to be given for more than a year and even then may not completely clear the infection, particularly infection of the toenails. Tablets are taken with food. Side effects are gastrointestinal disturbances and, less commonly, headaches, photosensitivity, and allergic reactions. The new oral antifungal agent terbinafine has produced promising results and will probably replace griseofulvin as the treatment of choice. Owing to its fungicidal action courses of two to three months are at least as effective as prolonged griseofulvin. Side effects reported so far are mild and limited to the gastrointestinal tract. Neither treatment is advised in pregnancy. Ketoconazole is another alternative and it needs to be given for the same length of time as griseofulvin. Liver toxicity has been reported and regular monitoring is necessary.

Other nail dystrophies

Psoriatic nail changes may improve if the general state of the skin improves. Potent topical steroids applied locally can produce some improvement but relapse is frequent.

Local eczematous disease—Changes related to a local eczematous process will gradually improve if the local skin remains clear.

Non-scarring lichen planus improves spontaneously. Progressive scarring may be helped by oral steroids. The nail changes of alopecia areata may persist after the hair loss has recovered. Treatment is unhelpful.

Local trauma—Problems related to local trauma, particularly chronic paronychia, lamellar splitting, and onycholysis, will improve if the underlying factors can be removed.

LUMPS AND BUMPS

The skin is a common site for neoplastic lesions, but most invade only locally and with treatment usually do not pose any threat to the life of the patient. The exception is malignant melanoma, which is dealt with in the next chapter. This is a rare tumour with a high mortality, and recent publicity campaigns have been aimed at preventing the tragedy of fatal metastases from a neglected melanoma.

As a result a large number of patients are being seen with pigmented skin lesions and nodules, only a very few of which are neoplastic. The question is how to distinguish the benign, the malignant, and the possibly malignant. The following guidelines may help in deciding whether the lesion can be safely left or should be treated.

A correlation of the clinical and pathological features is helpful in making a confident diagnosis of the more common tumours.

Seborrhoeic warts

Seborrhoeic warts come in various shapes, sizes, and colours. When deeply pigmented, inflamed, or growing they may appear to have the features of a malignant lesion, but the following features are characteristic.
- Well defined edge
- Warty, papillary surface—often with keratin plugs
- Raised above surrounding skin to give a "stuck on" appearance.

Individual lesions vary considerably in size, but are usually 0·5–3 cm in diameter. Protuberant and pedunculated lesions occur. Solitary lesions are commonly seen on the face and neck but more numerous, large lesions tend to occur on the trunk. They become more common with increasing age.

Basal cell carcinoma

In contrast, the early basal cell carcinoma—or rodent ulcer—presents as a firm nodule, clearly growing within the skin and below it, rather than on the surface. The colour varies from that of normal skin to dark brown or black, but there is commonly a "pearly" translucent quality. As its name implies, the tumour is composed of masses of dividing basal cells that have lost the capacity to differentiate any further. As a

Epidermis

Normal basal layer

Nodular basal cell carcinoma

Ulcerated basal cell carcinoma

Ulcer with a rolled edge

Becomes →

Clumps of neoplastic basal cells

Lumps and bumps

Cystic basal cell carcinoma.

Superficial basal cell carcinoma.

Pigmented basal cell carcinoma.

Neglected basal cell carcinoma (rodent ulcer).

result no epidermis is formed over the tumour and the surface breaks down to form an ulcer, the residual edges of the nodule forming the characteristic "rolled edge." Once the basal cells have invaded the deeper tissues the rolled edge disappears.

Variants

Variants of the usual pattern can cause problems in diagnosis. *Cystic* basal cell carcinomas occur and those that show differentiation towards hair follicles or sweat glands may have a less typical appearance. *Pigmented* lesions can resemble melanoma. The *superficial spreading* type may be confused with a patch of eczema. This usually occurs on the trunk, does not itch, and shows a gradual but inexorable increase in size. A firm "whipcord" edge may be present.

Treatment

Various methods of destroying tumour tissue are used and the results are similar for radiotherapy and surgical excision.

(1) Ulcerated lesions may invade tissue planes, blood vessels, and nerves more extensively than is clinically apparent.

(2) Although modern techniques of radiotherapy result in minimal scarring and atrophy these may cause problems near the eye.

(3) Basal cell carcinomas in skin creases, such as the nasolabial fold, tend to ulcerate and are hard to excise adequately.

(4) Surgical excision has the advantage that should the lesion recur radiotherapy is available to treat it, whereas it is not desirable to treat recurrences after radiotherapy with further irradiation.

Squamous cell carcinoma

Squamous cell carcinoma represents proliferation of the epidermal keratinocytes in a deranged manner—with a visible degree of differentiation into epidermal cells that may show individual cell keratinisation and "pearls" of keratin. In other tumours bizarre cells with mitoses, cells with clear cytoplasm, or spindle cells may be seen.

Squamous neoplastic cells

This type of cancer often develops at a site of previous damage to the skin—for example, from sunlight or chemical damage. The first change clinically is a thickening of the skin with scaling or hyperkeratosis of the surfaces. The more differentiated tumours often have a warty, keratotic crust while others may be nodular. The edge is poorly defined. There may be associated dilated, telangiectatic blood vessels. The original hard, disc like lesion becomes nodular and ulcerates with strands of tumour cells invading the deeper tissue. The thick warty crust, often found elsewhere, may be absent from the lesions on the lip, buccal mucosa, and penis.

These histological changes complement the clinical appearance and are clearly different from those of basal cell carcinoma.

Treatment—Small lesions should be excised as a rule, making sure that the palpable edge of the tumour is included, with a 3–5 mm margin. Radiotherapy is effective but fragile scars may be a disadvantage on the hand. Cryotherapy or topical fluorouracil can be used for histologically confirmed, superficial lesions and also for solar keratoses.

Solar keratoses

Squamous cell carcinoma may develop in solar keratoses, which show thickening of the epidermis and abnormal keratinocytes. They occur on sites exposed to the sun and are more common on those who have worked out of doors or sunbathed excessively. They can be regarded as squamous cell carcinomas grade 1/2 but do not necessarily progress to a dysplastic carcinoma. They also develop on the lips, particularly of pipe smokers.

The clinical appearance varies from a simple rough area of skin to a keratotic lesion with marked inflammation. The edge and surface are irregular.

Treatment with cryotherapy, using liquid nitrogen or carbon dioxide, repeated if necessary, is usually effective.

5-Fluorouracil cream is useful for larger or multiple lesions. It is applied twice daily for two weeks, which produces inflammation and necrosis. Simple dressings are applied for the next two weeks. This process can be repeated if necessary. As it is a cytotoxic drug it should be handled with care and applied sparingly with a cotton bud while wearing gloves.

Other conditions

Bowen's disease.

Bowen's disease is characterised by a well defined, erythematous macule with little induration and slight crusting. It is a condition of the middle aged and elderly, occurring commonly on the trunk and limbs. It is an intraepidermal carcinoma, which has been reported to follow the ingestion of arsenic in "tonics" taken in years gone by or exposure to sheep dip, weedkiller, or industrial processes. After many years florid carcinoma may develop with invasion of deeper tissues. It may be confused with a patch of eczema or superficial basal cell carcinoma. Lesions on covered areas may be associated with underlying malignancy. Erythroplasia of Queyrat is a similar process occurring on the glans penis or prepuce.

Paget's disease of the nipple.

Keratoacanthoma.

Paget's disease of the nipple presents with unilateral non-specific erythematous changes on the aureola and nipple, spreading to the surrounding skin. The cause is an underlying adenocarcinoma of the ducts. It should be considered in any patient with eczematous changes of one breast that fail to respond to simple treatment. Extramammary lesions occur.

Keratoacanthoma is a rapidly growing fleshy nodule that develops a hard keratotic centre. Healing occurs with some scarring. Although benign, it may recur after being removed with curette and cautery, particularly from the face, and is best excised.

Benign tumours

Dermatofibroma (top left), skin tags (above), and syringoma (left).

Dermatofibroma—This is a simple, discrete firm nodule, arising in the dermis at the site of an insect bite or other trivial injury. Often there is a brown or red vascular lesion initially which then becomes fibrotic—a sclerosing haemangioma. The histiocytoma is similar but composed of histiocytes.

Skin tags may be pigmented but rarely cause any diagnostic problems unless inflamed. Some are in fact pedunculated seborrhoeic warts and others simple papillomas (fibroepithelial polyps).

Other benign tumours

A wide variety of tumours may develop from the hair follicle and sebaceous, exocrine (sweat), and apocrine glands. The more common include *syringomas*—slowly growing, small, multiple nodules on the face of eccrine gland origin.

Lumps and bumps

Verrucous epidermal naevus.

Naevus sebaceous.

Epidermoid cyst.

Milia.

Naevus sebaceous is warty, well defined, varying in size from a small nodule to one several centimetres in diameter. Lesions occur in the scalp of children, may be present at birth, and gradually increase in size. They may proliferate or develop into a basal cell carcinoma in adult life and they are therefore best removed.

Verrucous epidermal naevi are probably a variant, found on the trunk and limbs.

Cysts

The familiar *epidermoid cyst*—also known as sebaceous cyst or wen—occurs as a soft, well defined, mobile swelling usually on the face, neck, shoulder, and chest. It is not derived from sebaceous glands but contains keratin produced by the lining wall.

Pilar cysts on the scalp are similar lesions derived from hair follicles.

Milia are small keratin cysts consisting of small white papules found on the cheek and eyelids.

Vascular lesions

Naevus flammeus.

Sturge-Weber syndrome.

The more common vascular naevi are mentioned.

The port wine stain, or naevus flammeus, presents at birth as a flat red lesion, usually on the face, neck, or upper trunk. There is usually a sharp midline border on the more common unilateral lesions. In time the affected area becomes raised and thickened because of proliferation of vascular and connective tissue. If the area supplied by the ophthalmic or maxillary divisions of the trigeminal nerve is affected there may be associated angiomas of the underlying meninges with epilepsy—Sturge-Weber syndrome. Lesions of the limb may be associated with arteriovenous fistulae.

Cavernous angioma
in a 5 months old baby.

Five years later.

Cavernous angioma—strawberry naevi—appear in the first few weeks of life or at birth. A soft vascular swelling is found, most commonly on the head and neck. The lesions resolve spontaneously in time and do not require treatment.

Spider naevi.

Pyogenic granuloma.

Spider naevus consist of a central vascular papule with fine lines radiating from it. They are more common in children and women. Large numbers in a man raise the possibility of liver disease.

Campbell de Morgan spots are discrete red papules 1–5 mm in diameter. They are more common on the trunk.

Pyogenic granuloma is a lesion that contains no pus but is in fact vascular and grows rapidly. It may arise at the site of trauma. Distinction from amelanotic melanoma is important.

BLACK SPOTS IN THE SKIN

There has been a great increase in public awareness of melanoma and any dark lesions of the skin are sometimes regarded with the same dread as Long John Silver's "black spot" in *Treasure Island*—a sign of imminent demise. However, the vast majority of pigmented lesions are simply moles or harmless pigmented naevi. The most important thing is to know which moles can be safely ignored and which should be removed. Benign moles are described first, then malignant melanoma, followed by a discussion of the differences between these two.

Benign moles

Benign pigmented naevi. Blue naevus

Spitz naevus.

Congenital hairy naevus.

Halo naevus. Dysplastic naevus syndrome.

Becker's naevus.

Benign moles are naevi with a proliferation of melanocytes and a variable number of dermal naevus cells. Most develop in early childhood and adolescence. The number of moles remains constant during adult life with a gradual decrease from the sixth decade onwards.

There is often an increase in both the number of moles and the degree of pigmentation during pregnancy.

Acquired melanocytic naevi

Acquired melanocytic naevi are the familiar moles and present in a number of different ways depending on the type of cells and the depth in the skin.

Junctional naevi are flat macules with melanocytes proliferating along the dermo-epidermal border.

Compound naevi have pigmented naevus cells at the dermo-epidermal border and in the dermis, producing a raised brown lesion. The dermal melanocytes may accumulate around the skin appendages and blood vessels and form a band of cells without melanin or more deeply penetrating strands of spindle cells. Proliferating naevus cells may throw the overlying epidermis into folds, giving a papillary appearance.

In a purely *intradermal naevus* the junctional element is lost, with the deeper cells showing characteristics of neural tissue. Other types of acquired pigmented naevi include:

Blue naevus—This is a collection of deeply pigmented melanocytes situated deep in the dermis, which accounts for the deep slate-blue colour.

Spitz naevus—This presents as a fleshy pink papule in chidren. It is composed of large spindle cells and epitheloid cells with occasional giant cells, arranged in "nests." It is benign and the old name of juvenile melanoma should be abandoned.

Halo naevus—This consists of a melanocytic naevus with a surrounding halo of depigmentation associated with the presence of antibodies against melanocytes in some cases. The whole naevus gradually fades in time.

Becker's naevus—This is an area of increased pigmentation, often associated with increased hair growth, which is usually seen on the upper trunk or shoulders. It is benign.

Freckles or ephelides—These are small pigmented macules, less than 0.5 cm in diameter, that occur in areas exposed to the sun in fair skinned people then fade during the winter months.

Dysplastic naevus syndrom—Multiple pigmented naevi occur, predominantly on the trunk, becoming numerous during adolescence. They vary in size—many being over 0·5 cm—and tend to develop malignant melanoma, particularly if there is a family history of this condition.

Congenital pigmented naevi

Congenital pigmented naevi are present at birth, generally over 1 cm in diameter, and vary from pale brown to black in colour. They often become hairy and more protuberant, possibly with an increased risk of malignant change. Larger lesions can cover a considerable area of the trunk and buttocks, such as the bathing trunk naevi, and their removal may present a considerable problem.

Melanoma

Melanoma is an invasive malignant tumour of melanocytes. Most cases occur in white adults over the age of 30, with a predominance in women.

Incidence—The incidence of melanoma has doubled over the past 10 years in Australia (currently 40/100 000 population) and shown a similar increase in other countries. In Europe twice as many women as men develop melanoma—about 12/100 000 women and 6/100 000 men.

Prognosis—The prognosis is related to the thickness of the lesion, measured histologically in millimetres from the granular layer to the deepest level of invasion. Lesions less than 0.76 mm thick have a 100% survival at five years, 0.76–1.5 mm thick an 80% survival at five years, and lesions over 3.5 mm less than 40% survival. These figures are based on patients in whom the original lesion had been completely excised. A recent study in Scotland has shown an overall five year survival of 71.6%–77.6% for women and 58.7% for men.

Sun exposure—The highest incidence of melanoma occurs in countries with the most sunshine throughout the year. However, skin type and the regularity of exposure to sun are also important. The incidence is much greater in fair skinned people from higher latitudes who have concentrated exposure to sun during holidays than those with darker complexions who have more regular exposure throughout the year. Severe sunburn may also predispose to melanoma.

Nodular melanoma.

Superficial melanoma with nodules.

Lentigo maligna.

Genetic factors—Since melanin protects the skin from ultraviolet light it is not surprising that melanoma occurs most commonly in fair skinned people who show little tanning on exposure to sun, particularly those of celtic origin. Members of families with the dysplastic naevus syndrome are more likely to develop melanoma in their moles. These patients have multiple naevi from a young age.

Pre-existing moles—It is rare for ordinary moles to become malignant but congenital naevi and multiple dysplastic naevi are more likely to develop into malignant melanoma.

Types of melanoma

There are four main types of melanoma.

Superficial spreading melanoma is the more common variety. It is common on the back in men and on the legs in women. As the name implies the melanoma cells spread superficially in the epidermis, becoming invasive after months or years. The margin and the surface are irregular with pigmentation varying from brown to black. There may be surrounding inflammation and there is often clearing of the central portion. The invasive phase is associated with the appearance of nodules and increased pigmentation. The prognosis is correspondingly poor.

Nodule developing in superficial spreading melanoma.

Superficial spreading melanoma.

Acral melanoma.

Lentigo maligna melanoma occurs characteristically in areas exposed to sun in elderly people. Initially there is a slowly growing, irregular pigmented macule that is present for many years before a melanoma develops.

Nodular melanoma presents as a dark nodule from the start without a preceding in situ epidermal phase. It is more common in men than women and is usually seen in people in their 50s and 60s. Because it is a vertical invasive growth phase from the beginning there is a poor prognosis.

Nodular melanoma in a lentigo.

Talon noir.

Benign lentigo.

Dysplastic melanoma.

Amelanotic melanoma.

Malignant melanoma in a black person. Note the surrounding "halo."

Acral melanoma occurs on the palm and soles and near or under the nails. Benign pigmented naevi may also occur in these sites and it is important to recognise early dysplastic change by using the criteria set out below. A very important indication that discoloration of the nail is due to melanoma is Hutchinson's sign—pigmentation of the nail fold adjacent to the nail. It is important to distinguish *talon noir*, in which a black area appears on the sole or heel. It is the result of trauma—for example, sustained while playing squash—causing haemorrhage into the dermal papillae. Paring the skin gently with a scalpel will reveal distinct blood filled papillae, to the relief of doctor and patient alike.

Other types of melanoma—As the melanoma cells become more dysplastic and less well differentiated they lose the capacity to produce melanin and form an *amelanonitic melanoma*. Such non-pigmented nodules may be regarded as harmless but are in fact extremely dangerous.

How to tell the difference

> ### Criteria for suspecting malignant changes in pigmented lesions
>
> (1) *Growth*—Benign pigmented naevi continue to appear in adolescents and young adults. Any mole increasing in size in an adult over the age of 30 may be a melanoma
>
> (2) *Shape*—Moles usually have a symmetrical, even outline, any indentations being quite regular; melanomas usually have an irregular edge with one part advancing more than the others
>
> (3) *Colour*—Variation in colour of benign moles is even but a melanoma may be intensely black or show irregular colouration varying from white to slate blue, with all shades of black and brown. Inflammation may give a red colour as well. The amelanotic melanoma shows little or no pigmentation
>
> (4) *Size*—Apart from congenital pigmentation naevi most benign moles are less than 1 cm in diameter. Any lesion growing to over 0.5 cm should be carefully checked
>
> (6) *Itching*—normally a mole does not itch but a melanoma may. Irritated seborrhoeic warts also itch
>
> (7) *Bleeding* and crusting occur in an actively growing melanoma
>
> **If more than two of these features are present refer the patient for specialist opinion**
>
> *A simple summary:*
>
> A—**A**symmetry of the lesion   B—Irregularity of the **B**order
> C—Variations in **C**olour   D—**D**iameter larger than 0.5 cm

Benign moles show little change and remain static for years. Any change may indicate that a mole is in fact a melanoma or that a mole is becoming active. Size, shape, and colour are the most significant features and it is *change* in them that is most important. Patients with moles should have these changes explained to them, in particular that they indicate activity of the cells, not necessarily malignant change.

The sun and the skin

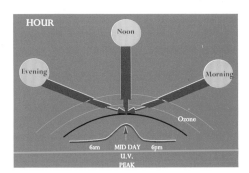

There is general awareness that the sun causes cancer in the skin with some people becoming obsessively fearful of any exposure to sun. A sensible approach with emphasis on reasonable precautions is called for. Useful points are:

- The non-melanotic, epidermal cancers—basal cell and squamous cell carcinomas—grow slowly and are not life threatening. Exposure to sun has usually occurred many years previously
- Most moles are entirely harmless
- Detecting the changes in moles or early melanoma, as outlined above, enables the diagnosis to be made at an early stage with a good chance of curative treatment
- Good sunscreen preparations should be used when outside in strong sunlight
- Reflected sun from the sea or beach can be nearly as damaging as direct sunlight
- Exposure to midday sun, particularly in tropical or subtropical latitudes, should be avoided. At this time the sunlight passes vertically through the atmosphere and there is less filtering of dangerous ultraviolet light.

PRACTICAL PROCEDURES

D W S Harris

Skin biopsy

Many common conditions can successfully be dealt with by simple techniques which, once acquired, can easily be used in general practice. In this chapter several of the most useful are discussed.

Skin biopsy is used to establish a diagnosis (incisional) or to remove a lesion (excisional). In both cases the incision should be elliptical and should run parallel to the skin wrinkle lines.

As a rule of thumb the long axis of the wound should be about three times as long as its short axis. The apical angle should be no more than 30°.

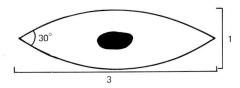

Procedure

(1) Explain the procedure to the patient, warning about the scar that will result from it. This may be slight on the face but more prominent in areas susceptible to keloid formation, such as the sternum, shoulders, and upper outer arms.

(2) Establish that the patient is not allergic to local anaesthetics.

(3) Obtain consent.

(4) Mark out the planned incision with sterile gentian violet before injecting the local anaesthetic.

(5) Anaesthetise with 1–2% plain lignocaine. Lignocaine-adrenaline combinations, though they help to reduce bleeding, should not be used on the extremities for fear of ischaemic damage. The mild discomfort of the injection may be lessened by injecting very slowly and avoiding lignocaine-adrenaline mixtures. Warming the anaesthetic diminishes the pain of injection.

(6) A number 15 blade is used, cutting at 90° to the skin surface. Wedge shaped incisions heal poorly, as illustrated.

(7) A skin hook may be used to lift one end of the specimen to release its underside. Toothed forceps may crush the specimen and cause pathological artefacts.

(8) Removal of sutures—from the face at 4–5 days, from the trunk at 7–14 days, and from the leg at 10–14 days.

(9) Elevation and compression bandaging are advisable when removing lesions from the lower leg.

Normal Abnormal Normal Abnormal

Clinical. Surgical. Histopathological.

Incisional biopsy—Always include the boundary of the normal-abnormal area in an incisional biopsy specimen, which must be at least 1 cm long and deep enough to include subcutaneous tissue.

Excisional biopsy—There are several points to remember when removing a lesion.

(1) Allow for an adequate zone of clearance, especially when excising pigmented or neoplastic lesions. A 2·5–5 mm margin is usually sufficient. Partial removal must be avoided.

(2) Place secimens, dermal side down, on a small square of filter paper, to avoid curling, and then immerse them in formalin.

(3) Mark clearly on the specimen container the patient's name and the date of biopsy.

(4) Record on the pathology form the site of biopsy, a description of the lesion and a note of its duration, the clinical history, and the clinical diagnosis.

Curettage

Seborrhoeic keratosis. Actinic keratosis.

Curettage is ideal for benign epidermal lesions, such as seborrhoeic and actinic keratoses or viral warts.

If well localised on the face, trunk, and limbs superficial or small nodulocystic basal cell carcinomas may be treated by curettage if they have clearcut borders and a firm base. Such specimens must be sent for histological confirmation and the scars reviewed regularly.

Procedure

(1) Anaesthetise site.

(2) Stretch the skin on either side of the lesion.

(3) Apply the lip of the curette to the edge of the lesion, as illustrated.

(4) Use a rapid downward scooping action, working around the lesion towards its centre.

(5) Curette down to the dermis, identifiable by its scratchy, sandpaper-like consistency.

(6) Use light cautery, sweeping across the base of the lesion, and pay particular attention to bleeding points. Necrotic tissue produced by excessive cautery impairs wound healing: simple pressure to control bleeding is preferable to this.

(7) Repeat the whole procedure if treating a basal cell carcinoma.

(8) Cover with a dry dressing on the trunk: leave facial lesions exposed. Tell the patient that a scab will form and drop off in about 10 days.

Cryotherapy

Applying the liquid nitrogen.

Cryotherapy is used increasingly to treat many dermatological conditions in hospital and general practice. Suitable conditions include (*a*) viral warts and molluscum contagiosum; (*b*) keratoses, both seborrhoeic and actinic; and (*c*) biopsy proved Bowen's disease. Local anaesthetic is usually not needed.

A liqid nitrogen spray may be used but equally good results can be obtained with a cottonwool dipstick method. The best results are then achieved by "rolling your own." After immersing the cottonwool bud in liquid nitrogen apply it firmly to the lesion.

Practical procedures

The frozen wart.

Subsequent slight blistering.

Wait until a thin "halo" of frozen tissue has spread 2 mm out from the base of the lesion. Depending on size, this usually takes 5 to 10 seconds.

Repeat once if necessary.

Precautions

(1) Take great care with lesions on the faces of children and with pigmented skins. Hypopigmentation and hyperpigmentation can occur.

(2) Treat only if the diagnosis is certain: a confirmatory biopsy may be needed before treatment—as in Bowen's disease.

(3) Warn that a haemorrhagic blister may form at the site within 24 hours. This tendency can be reduced by a single application of a highly potent corticosteroid ointment immediately after treatment. Should a blister form it will remain for several days. If it is painful a sterile needle may be used to burst it and then a dry dressing can be applied.

(4) It may be unwise to treat lesions on both hands or feet at the same visit as having both hands or both feet with painful lesions could interfere with daily activitities.

Electrocautery

A heated element is used to coagulate the lesions. As no current passes through the body this is a safe procedure.

Common indications include (*a*) the removal of benign epidermal pedunculated tumours, such as skin tags; and (*b*) the destruction of small vascular lesions such as spider naevi. Only lesions that need no histological confirmation should be treated. Other indications for this procedure lie outside the scope of this article. There are two modes of cautery—shave cautery and pinpoint cautery.

Shave cautery is used on skin tags over 1 cm long. The correct attachment is needed. Pick up the skin tag with forceps and slice across the base with the cautery instrument. Local anaesthetic may be required.

Equally well tolerated is touching a skin tag with the needle or ball point tip directly. The lesion mummifies immediately and drops off in 10 days.

Smaller lesions may be simply snipped off.

Pinpoint cautery attachment.

Blanch the lesion to identify feeding vessels. Then insert needle into feeding vessels in the cold state.

Spider naevus.

Pinpoint cautery is used on lesions such as spider naevi. A pinpoint attachment is needed. Locate the feeding vessel by blanching with a glass slide. Accurately position the needle element in the cold state into the lesion and apply current for less than 1 second. Warn the patient that a small scab will develop and fall off within 10 days. A local anaesthetic is seldom needed.

AUTOIMMUNITY AND SKIN DISEASE

D J Gawkrodger

Hypersensitivity

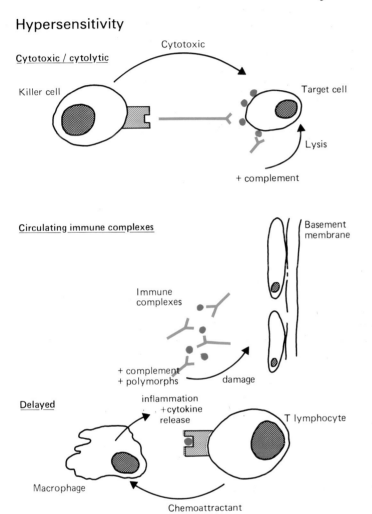

Autoimmunity is the state where the normal mechansims of tolerance to self antigens are broken down. Autoantibodies and autoantigen specific T lymphocytes develop.

Autoantibodies may be produced against an organ specific antigen—for example, bullous pemphigoid antigen—or against a very widely distributed antigen such as DNA, as in lupus erythematosus. Not surprisingly, the resulting disease can be organ specific or non-organ specific. The pathogenesis is complex. It is not simply the effect of T lymphocytes locking on to autoantibody coated target cells with subsequent cell death ("cytotoxic" hypersensitivity); damage due to the deposition of circulating immune complexes; or, in some instances, cell mediated ("delayed") hypersensitivity related to specifically sensitised T cells and their release of cytokines (molecules that mediate actions between cells). Defects in the control of immunological tolerance by T suppressor cells are now thought to be implicated as well.

Autoimmune diseases often run in families. Individuals with certain human leucocyte antigen (HLA) haplotypes are well known to be at risk of developing Hashimoto's thyroiditis or pernicious anaemia, and the same is true for systemic lupus erythematosus and pemphigus.

The skin reflects the range of autoimmune disease

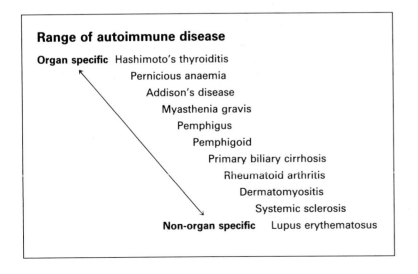

The skin is often an indicator of internal conditions, and autoimmunity is no exception. Pigmentation accompanies some organ specific disorders, such as Hashimoto's thyroiditis, Addison's disease, and primary biliary cirrhosis. A lemon yellow hue and canities occur with pernicious anaemia, and vitiligo like lesions and alopecia areata may be found in individuals with various autoimmune problems.

Non-organ specific autoimmune diseases often have prominent skin disease—for example, lupus erythematosus, systemic sclerosis, and dermatomyositis—but there are cutaneous organ specific disorders, principally pemphigus and pemphigoid.

Autoimmunity and skin disease

Pemphigoid

Split at dermatoepidermal junction.

Usually a condition of the elderly with a slight preponderance among women, bullous pemphigoid is characterised by large tense blisters arising on erythematous or normal looking skin. The limbs, trunk, and flexures are commonly affected; mouth lesions occur in 10% of patients. The disease responds readily to modest doses of oral prednisolone, and spontaneous remission is seen in up to half of subjects, although relapses may occur.

Direct immunofluorescence.

Fluorescein labelled antibody to human immunoglobulin

Antibody (immunoglobulin) in situ

Normal antigen

Skin section from patient

Indirect immunofluorescence.

Fluorescein labelled antibody to human immunoglobulin

Antibody in patient's serum, placed on section

Antigen similar to human

Substrate (usually animal tissue)

Histologically, the blisters are subepidermal. Most patients have antibodies directed against the basement membrane zone circulating in their blood. These antibodies, usually of the IgG type, may be identified in serum by the *indirect* immunofluorescence method. This uses a tissue substrate (animal or sometimes human skin) cut freshly as a thin section on a slide, on to which the patient's serum is applied; the antibodies which attach to the basement membrane zone are shown by subsequently applying an antihuman immunoglobulin antibody which has been tagged with fluorescein, so that it shows up when the slide is visualised under ultraviolet radiation. The anti-basement membrane zone antibodies can be shown in a patient's perilesional skin by *direct* immunofluorescence. A freshly cut section of skin is reacted with a fluorescein labelled antibody to human IgG, and the deposited IgG can be seen as a continuous band at the basement membrane zone. The anti-BMZ antibodies are directed against bullous pemphigoid antigen, located in the hemidesmosome at the basement membrane zone, and synthesised by the basal cells of the epidermis. The pemphigoid autoantibodies have an indirect effect: they activate complement and attract inflammatory cells. Lysosomal enzymes are released which damage the basement membrane and result in blistering.

Other types of pemphigoid, such as cicatricial (which affects the ocular or oral membranes) or "localised" (often affecting a limited area on the head or neck), show similar histological and immunofluorescence profiles, although circulating anti-basement membrane zone antibodies are less commonly found. The same applies for pemphigoid ("herpes") gestationis, a rare but characteristic bullous eruption of pregnancy.

Indirect immunofluorescence.

Pemphigus

Less common than pemphigoid and more likely to prove fatal, pemphigus vulgaris is a disease of middle life. Oral lesions signal the onset in half of the patients and often precede cutaneous disease by months. Fragile superficial bilisters develop over the scalp, face, back, chest, and flexures: the bullous element may not be apparent and lesions may consist of crusted erosions. Unlike with pemphigoid, high doses of prednisolone (often with other immunosuppressive agents) are required and spontaneous remission is exceptional.

The blister is intraepidermal. Ninety per cent of patients have circulating autoantibodies, IgG in type, directed against an intercellular substance of the epidermis and identifiable by indirect immunofluorescence. The levels of these antibodies correlate with disease activity. The antigen responsible has been localised to the desmosome of the keratinocyte. Antibodies bind to this antigen and stimulate the production of plasmin from plasminogen. Plasmin induces loss of cell to cell adhesion and an intraepidermal split results. Direct immunofluorescence shows IgG antibodies deposited on the intercellular substance of the suprabasal epidermis in almost all patients.

Intraepidermal split.

Direct immunofluorescence.

Other variants of pemphigus exist. Pemphigus vegetans gives hypertrophic, papillomatous lesions, whereas pemphigus foliaceus is characterised by shallow erosions on the face and scalp, and pemphigus erythematosus has some features of lupus erythematosus. Pemphigus is sometimes associated with myasthenia gravis, another organ specific autoimmune disease. Treatment with penicillamine or captopril can induce pemphigus: the eruption usually resolves when treatment with the drug is stopped.

Alopecia areata and vitiligo

Alopecia areata.

Organ specific autoimmune diseases are more prevalent than expected in patients with both vitiligo and alopecia areata, and afflicted patients have an increased prevalence of organ specific autoantibodies. Despite these associations there is little direct evidence as yet to implicate alopecia areata or vitiligo as an autoimmune disease. However, some patients with vitiligo seem to have antibodies to melanocytes and the numbers of helper T cells may be decreased, and in alopecia areata T cell regulation may be impaired.

Lupus erythematosus

Clinical variants of lupus erythematosus

Systemic
Subacute cutaneous
Discoid
(Neonatal)

Discoid lupus erythematosus and systemic lupus erythematosus seem to be variants of the same disease, although only about 5% of those with the discoid type progress to systemic disease. A variety of autoantibodies to nuclear, nucleolar, and cytoplasmic antigens are found in lupus erythematosus. Almost 90% of patients with systemic lupus erythematosus have circulating antinuclear antibodies, but only a third of those with discoid lupus erythematosus show circulating antibodies.

Three quarters of patients with systemic lupus erythematosus have cutaneous disease. The "butterfly" eruption over the face is well known, but other cutaneous signs include photosensitivity, discoid lesions, alopecia, and vasculitis. A diagnosis of systemic lupus erythematosus requires the demonstration of multisystem disease with serological or haematological abnormalities. In addition to circulating antibodies, direct immunofluorescence of skin where there are no lesions may show granular deposition of various immunoglobins and complement components at the dermoepidermal junction, the "lupus band" test.

In discoid lupus erythematosus, the discoid lesions typically occur in areas exposed to light, usually on the face. Circulating antinuclear antibodies and systemic symptoms are infrequent, although the "lupus band" test may be positive in lesional skin.

Patients with "subacute cutaneous" lupus erythematosus have a distinctive annular eruption, often with systemic (but not renal) disease, and usually show circulating antibodies to a cytoplasmic RNA nucleotide (Ro). Anti-Ro antibodies are similarly found in neonatal lupus erythematosus, which also has definitive skin signs.

Lupus erythematosus is often thought of as an immune complex disease with defects in T suppressor cell function. Ultraviolet radiation may generate antigenic nuclear products in the skin, with the development of clinical disease.

Subacute lupus erythematosus.

Discoid lupus erythematosus.

Dermatomyositis

The dermatomyositis-polymyositis complex is a heterogeneous group of disorders with varying involvement of skin and muscle. Associations with malignancy, particularly in men aged over 40, and connective tissue disease, especially rheumatoid arthritis and systemic lupus erythematosus, represent distinct subtypes.

The purplish red heliotrope erythema around the eyelids, cheeks, and forehead, often with oedema, is typical. Bluish red scaly plaques on the dorsal aspects of the fingers and hands (especially over the joints) and nail fold telangiectasia are other features, although the eruption can be widespread.

Abnormalities of humoral and cellular immunity suggest an autoimmune cause. Although not specific, antibodies to skeletal muscle are found, and lymphocytes from affected patients show enhanced transformation on exposure to muscle antigens. Deposits of IgG, IgM, or C3 are described in skeletal muscle blood vessels on direct immunofluorescence, and IgG or IgM may be seen in the upper dermis. Antinuclear antibodies and circulating immune complexes are present in the serum of some subjects.

Systemic sclerosis and morphoea

Systemic sclerosis.   Morphoea.

Morphoea, localised plaques or bands of sclerotic skin, is clinically distinct from systemic sclerosis, though histologically the skin changes are similar. Morphoea is a local form of systemic sclerosis, but affected patients lack the serological characteristics of the latter, and internal disease is uncommon or mild.

Skin changes are prominent in systemic sclerosis. Raynaud's phenomenon is almost invariable: the skin of the hands and forearms becomes tight and waxy, with atrophy of the finger pulp and flexion deformities. Telangiectasia, with radial furrowing around the mouth and restricted mouth opening, are characteristic. Disease of internal organs must be expected.

Almost all patients with systemic sclerosis have antibodies to nuclear or cytoplasmic antigens in their serum samples and 50% have circulating immune complexes. Endothelial cell damage, related to humoral or T cell derived factors, may initiate a cascade of inflammation which results in fibrosis and sclerosis of the target organ.

Graft versus host disease

Graft versus host disease occurs after bone marrow transplantation, when immunocompetent cells of the graft react against the histoincompatible tissues of the immunosuppressed recipient. Activated T cells release cytokines, activating cytotoxic cells which attack the epidermis and other tissues. Acute and chronic forms are recognised, with cutaneous changes including a morbilliform eruption, toxic epidermal necrolysis, a lichen planus like eruption, and a scleroderma like syndrome. In chronic graft versus host disease immunoglobulins and complement proteins are found in the walls of dermal blood vessels.

Lichen sclerosus

Lichen sclerosus or "white spot disease" is an uncommon condition that affects 10 times more women than men. There is an increased prevalence of autoimmune disorders and organ specific autoantibodies in those with the disease. Lichen sclerosus in women takes the form of ivory white wrinkled plaques on the vulva and perineum. In men the condition is also known as balanitis xerotica obliterans and appears as shiny bluish-white sclerotic areas on the glans penis and foreskin, which may produce phimosis. Squamous cell carcinoma is a potential complication in both sexes. Extragenital lesions may occur. Children are occasionally affected and tend to have a better prognosis than adults.

THE SKIN AND SYSTEMIC DISEASE

When a man has on the skin of his body a swelling or an eruption or a spot . . . and the disease appears to be deeper than the skin it is a leprous disease.

Leviticus 13:2-3

Although arguments continue about what the Old Testament writers understood by "leprous," there was clearly an appreciation of the connection between the skin and systemic illness. As in ancient times, clinical signs in the skin may give valuable diagnostic clues to underlying disease. Sometimes the same condition affects both the skin and other organs, or severe skin disease itself may be the cause of generalised illness.

The skin is also a common target organ for allergic reactions to drugs, with a rash being the first clinical sign. The florid skin lesions of AIDS illustrate the results of infections when the immune response is impaired.

The cutaneous signs of systemic disease is a very large subject, on which much has been written, so the presence of a skin eruption that might indicate systemic disease is good reason to consult the large textbooks. Nevertheless, it is possible to give an outline of the more common skin changes that may be associated with systemic illness.

Erythematous rashes

Rash from penicillin.   Erythema multiforme.

Allergic reactions to drugs, commonly the penicillins—There may be a widespread rash developing from a few days to two weeks after treatment with moderate illness (type III) or an acute life threatening anaphylactic reaction (types I and III) with acute angio-oedema and renal failure.

Infection—The characteristic rash of the various viral infections is, in a broad sense, also an allergic response. Less specific reactions such as erythema multiforme are commonly associated with infection—for example, herpes and other viral infections and streptococcal infection—but also with connective tissue disease and drugs such as sulphonamides.

In *carcinoid and phaeochromocytoma* vasoactive substances cause episodes of flushing and telangectasia.

Figurate erythema.   Erythema of nailbeds.

Dermatomyositis.

Neoplasia—Numerous patterns of widespread erythema have been described—the *"figurate erythemas"*—which may be associated with underlying carcinoma. *Dermatomyositis*, also a rare condition, has very high association in adults with underlying carcinoma commonly of the breasts, lung, ovary, or gastrointestinal tract. It is characterised by localised erythema with a purple hue, predominantly on the eyelids, cheeks, and forehead. There may be similar changes on the dorsal surface of the fingers often with dilated nail fold capillaries. These changes may precede the discovery of an underlying tumour and may also fade away once it is removed. There is variable association with muscle aching and weakness.

Erythema of the nailbeds may be associated with connective tissue disease—such as lupus erythematosus, scleroderma, and dermatomyositis. "Clubbing" of the fingers may be associated.

The skin and systemic disease

CREST syndrome.

Vasculitis.

Telangiectasia and clubbing may be features of scleroderma in the CREST syndrome. In this type of scleroderma there are **C**alcium deposits below the skin on the fingers and toes, **R**aynaud's phenomenon with poor peripheral circulation immobility of the o**E**sophagus, dermal **S**clerosis of the fingers and toes, and **T**elangiectasia of the face and lips and adjacent to the toe and finger nails.

Erythrocyanosis is a dusky, red, cyanotic change in the skin over the legs and thighs, where there is a deep layer of underlying fat. The condition becomes worse in the winter months. It is most common in young women and usually resolves over the years. Lupus erythematosus, sarcoidosis, and tuberculous infection may localise in affected areas.

Livedo reticularis is a cyanotic, net-like discoloration of the skin over the legs. It may be idiopathic or associated with arteritis or changes in blood viscosity.

Spider naevi, which show a central blood vessel with radiating branches, are frequently seen in women (especially during pregancy) and children. If they occur in large numbers, particularly in men, they may indicate liver failure. Palmar erythema and yellow nails may also be present.

Vasculitis and purpura of the skin may be associated with disease of the kidneys and other organs, as has already been discussed. "Splinter haemorrhages" under the nails are usually the result of minor trauma but may be associated with a wide range of conditions, including subacute bacterial endocarditis and rheumatoid arthritis.

Changes in pigmentation

Vitiligo.

Autoimmune associations with vitiligo

Thyroid disease	Myasthenia gravis
Pernicious anaemia	Alopecia areata
Hypoparathyroidism	Halo naevus
Addison's disease	Morphoea and
Diabetes	lichen sclerosus

Hypopigmentation

A widespread partial loss of melanocyte functions wih loss of skin colour is seen in hypopituitarism and is caused by an absence of melanocyte stimulating hormone. In the various types of autosomal recessive albinism there is a very considerable loss of pigment from the skin, hair, and eyes.

Localised depigmentation is most commonly seen in vitiligo, in which a family history of the condition is found in one third of the patients. In the sharply demarcated, symmetrical macular lesions there is loss of melanocytes and melanin. There is an increased incidence of organ specific antibodies and their associated diseases (table).

Other causes of hypopigmented macules include: postinflammatory conditions following psoriasis, eczema, lichen planus, and lupus erythematosus; infections—for example, tinea versicolor and leprosy; chemicals, such as hydroquinones, hydroxychloroquine, and arsenicals; reactions to pigmented naevi, seen in halo naevus; and genetic diseases, such as tuberous sclerosis ("ash leaf" macules).

Argyria (silver salts in skin).

Melasma.

Hyperpigmentation

There is wide variation in the pattern of normal pigmentation as a result of heredity and exposure to the sun. Darkening of the skin may be due to an increase in the normal pigment melanin or to the deposition of bile salts in liver disease, iron salts (haemochromatosis), drugs, or metallic salts from ingestion.

Causes of hyperpigmentation include the following.

Hormonal—An increase in circulating hormones that have melanocyte stimulating activity occurs in hyperthyroidism, Addison's disease, and acromegaly. In women who are pregnant or taking oral contraceptives there may be an increase in melanocytic pigmentation of the face. This is known as melasma (or chloasma) and occurs mainly on the forehead and cheeks. It may fade slowly. Sometimes a premenstrual darkening of the face occurs.

Increased deposition of haemosiderin is generalised in haemochromatosis. Localised red-brown discoloration of the legs is seen with longstanding varicose veins. It also occurs in a specific localised pattern in Schamberg's disease, when there is a "cayenne pepper" appearance of the legs and thighs.

Acanthosis nigricans.

Pseudoacanthosis nigricans.

Neoplasia—Lymphomas may be associated with increased pigmentation. *Acanthosis nigricans*, characterised by darkening and thickening of the skin of the axillae, neck, nipples, and umbilicus, occurs with internal cancers, usually adenocarcinoma of the stomach. It is also seen in acromegally. There is a benign juvenile type. *Pseudo acanthosis nigricans* is much more common, consisting of simple darkening of the skin in the flexures of obese individuals; it is not associated with malignancy.

Drugs—Chlorpromazine, other phenothiazines, and minocycline may cause an increased pigmentation in areas exposed to the sun. Phenytoin can cause local hyperpigmentation of the face and neck.

Inflammatory reactions—Post inflammatory pigmentation is common, often following acute eczema, fixed drug eruptions, or lichen planus. Areas of lichenification from rubbing the skin are commonly darkened.

Malabsorption and deficiency states—In malabsorption syndromes, pellagra, and scurvy there is commonly increased skin pigmentation.

Congenital conditions—There is clearly a marked variation in pigmentation and in the number of freckles in normal individuals. There may be localised well defined pigmented areas in neurofibromatosis with "cafe au lait" patches. Increased pigmentation with a blue tinge occurs over the lumbosacral region in the condition known as Mongolian blue spot.

Neurofibromatosis.

Peutz-Jeghers syndrome.

Peutz-Jeghers syndrome is inherited as an autosomal dominant characterised by pigmented macules of the oral mucosal membranes, lips, and face that appear in infancy. Benign intestinal polyps, mainly in the ileum and jejunum, which very rarely become malignant, are associated with the condition.

The skin and systemic disease

Malignant lesions

Lymphoma.

B cell lymphoma.

Pavapsoriasis.

Poikiloderma.

Malignant lesions may cause skin changes such as acanthosis nigricans and dermatomyositis or produce secondary lesions. Lymphomas can arise in or invade the skin and pruritus may be associated with Hodgkin's disease.

Mycosis fungoides is a T cell lymphoma of cutaneous origin. Initially well demarcated erythematous plaques develop on covered areas with intense itching. In many cases there is a gradual progression to infiltrated lesions, nodules, and ulceration. In others the tumour may occur de novo or be preceded by generalised erythema.

Poikiloderma, in which there is telangiectasia, reticulate pigmentation, atrophy, and loss of pigment, may precede mycosis fungoides, but it is also seen after radiotherapy and in connective tissue diseases.

Parapsoriasis is a term used for well defined maculopapular erythematous lesions that occur in middle and old age. Some cases undoubtedly develop into mycosis fungoides and a biopsy specimen should be taken of any such fixed plaques that do not clear with topical steroids.

The gut and the skin

Early pyoderma gangrenosum.

Pyoderma gangrenosum.

Dermatitis herpetiformis.

Vasculitis of various kinds, periarteritis nodosa, connective tissue diseases such as scleroderma, and many metabolic diseases produce both cutaneous and gastrointestinal lesions. There are, however, some specific associations.

Dry skin, asteatosis, and itching, with superficial eczematous changes and a "crazy paving" pattern, occur in malabsorption and cachectic states. Increased pigmentation, brittle hair and nails may also be associated.

Pyoderma gangrenosum—An area of non-specific inflammation and pustules breaks down to form a necrotic ulcer with hypertrophic margins. There is an underlying vasculitis. There is a strong association with ulcerative colitis and also with Crohn's disease, rheumatoid arthritis, and other diseases with an altered immune response.

Dermatitis herpetiformis, which has already been discussed, is an intensely itching, chronic disorder with erythematous and blistering lesions on the trunk and limbs. It is more common in men than women. Most patients have a gluten sensitive enteropathy with some degree of villus atrophy. There is an associated risk of small bowel lymphoma.

Other conditions—Peutz-Jeghers syndrome, with intestinal polyposis, has already been mentioned, but there are other rare congenital disorders with connective tissue and vascular abnormalities that affect the gut, such as Ehlers-Danlos syndrome and pseudoxanthoma elasticum (arterial gastrointestinal bleeding), purpuric vasculitis (bleeding from gastrointestinal lesions), and neurofibromatosis (intestinal neurofibromas).

Crohn's disease (regional ileitis)—Perianal lesions and sinus formation in the abdominal wall often occur. Glossitis and thickening of the lips and oral mucosa and vasculitis may be associated.

Diabetes and the skin

Diabetic ulcer.

Necrobiosis lipoidica.

Granuloma annulare.

In diabetes the disturbances of carbohydrate-lipid metabolism, small blood vessel lesions, and neural involvement may be associated with skin lesions. The more common of these include the following.

Infection—Diabetic patients have an increased susceptibility to staphylococcal, coliform, and pseudomonal infection. *Candida albicans* infection is also more common in diabetics.

Vascular lesions—"Diabetic dermopathy," due to a microangiopathy, consists of erythematous papules which slowly resolve to leave a scaling macule on the limbs. Atherosclerosis with impaired peripheral circulation is often associated with diabetes.

Ulceration due to neuropathy (trophic ulcers) or impaired blood supply may occur, particularly on the feet.

Specific skin lesions

Necrobiosis lipoidica—40–60% of patients with this condition may develop diabetes but it is not very common in diabetic patients (0·3%). As the name indicates, there is necrosis of the connective tissue with lymphocytic and granulomatous infiltrate. There is replacement of degenerating collagen fibres with lipid material. It usually occurs over the shin but may appear at any site.

Granuloma annulare usually presents with localised papular lesions on the hands and feet but may occur elsewhere. The lesions may be partly or wholly annular and may be single or multiple. There is some degree of necrobiosis with histiocytes forming "palisades" as well as giant cells and lymphocytes. It is seen more commonly in women, usually those aged under 30. There is an association with insulin dependent diabetes. In itself it is a harmless and self limiting condition that slowly clears but may recur.

Other diseases

Porphyria.

Xanthomas.

Porphyrias are due to the accumulation of intermediate metabolites in the metabolic pathway of haem synthesis. There are several types. In hepatic porphyrias there is skin fragility leading to blisters from exposure to the sun or minor trauma. In erythropoietic and erythrohepatic photoporphyrias there is intense photosensitivity. They are sometimes associated with sensitivity to long wavelength ultraviolet light that penetrates window glass.

Xanthomas are due to the deposition of fat in connective tissue cells. They are commonly associated with hyperlipidaemia—either primary or secondary to diabetes, the nephrotic syndrome, hypothyroidism, or primary biliary cirrhosis. Four of the primary types are associated with an increased risk of atherosclerosis; type I is not. Diabetes may be associated with the eruptive type.

Necrotising fasciitis—An area of cellulitis that develops vesicles and necrosis of the skin may indicate much more extensive, life threatening necrosis of the deeper tissues. Urgent surgical debridement is indicated.

Common types of xanthoma

Clinical type	Association with hyperlipidaemia	
	Primary type	Secondary
Xanthelasma of the eyelids—yellow plaques	II (may be normal)	–
Tuberous nodules on elbows and knees	II, III	+
Eruptive—small yellow papules on buttocks and shoulders	I, III, IV, V	+
Plane—yellow macules, palmar creases involved, generalised (myeloma)	I, III	+
Tendons—swelling on fingers or ankle	II, III	+

The skin and systemic disease

Pregnancy

Polymorphic eruption.

Pemphigoid gestationis.

Pregnancy may be associated with pruritus, in which the skin appears normal in 15–20% of women (prunigo gestationis). It is generally more servere in the first trimester.

Polymorphic eruptions also present with pruritis with urticaria papules and plaques (the PUPP syndrome). It usually occurs on the abdomen in the third trimester and then becomes widespread. There may be a postpartrum flare up. It can be a distressing condition for the mother but the baby is not affected and it rarely recurs in subsequent pregancies. Topical steroids can be used, but systemic steroids should be avoided.

Pemphigoid gestationis is a rare disorder that may resemble PUPP initially but develops pemphoid like vesicles, spreading over the abdomen and thighs: autoantibodies to the basement membrane are present.

Sarcoidosis

Sarcoidosis of the skin appears in various forms—as papules, nodules, plaques, or large cyanotic lesions ("lupus pernio"). Erythema nodosum may be associated.

Thyroid disease

Hypothyroidism	Hyperthyroidism
Dry skin	Soft, thickened skin
Oedema of eyelids and hands	Pretibial myxoedema
Absence of sweating	Increased sweating (palms and soles)
Coarse, thin hair—loss of pubic, axillary, and eyebrow hair	Thinning of scalp hair
Pale "ivory" skin	Diffuse pigmentation
Brittle poorly growing nails	Rapidly growing nails
Purpura, bruising, and telangiectasia	Palmar erythema
	Facial flushing

Thyroid disease is associated with changes in the skin, which may sometimes be the first clinical signs. There may be evidence of the effect of altered concentrations of thyroxine on the skin, with changes in texture and hair growth. Associated increases in thyroid stimulating hormone concentration may lead to pretibial myxoedema. In autoimmune thyroid disease vitiligo and other autoimmune conditions may be present.

Systemic malignancy

Skin signs of malignant disease

- Secondary deposits
- Secondary hormonal effects
  — Acne (adrenal tumours)
  — Flushing (carcinoid)
  — Pigmentation
- Generalised pruritus (particularly lymphoma)

- Figurate erythema
- Superficial thrombophlebitis
- Dermatomyositis
- Acanthosis nigricans
- Various eruptive skin lesions seen in Gardeners and Bazex syndromes

Genetics and skin disease

The fault, dear Brutus, is not in our stars but in ourselves
SHAKESPEARE, *Julius Caesar, Act I Sc 2.*

The knowledge that there may be underlying inherited factors when external causes have been excluded often helps patients come to terms with chronic skin disease that is otherwise inexplicable.

The commonest skin diseases, psoriasis and eczema, tend to run in families, suggesting that genetic factors are involved. Evidence for this in psoriasis is the association with the presence of antigens of the histocompatibility complex HLA-CW6. Recently HLA associated genes on chromosome 6 have been identified. The fact that when one parent is affected a child has a 25% chance of developing the disease suggests an autosomal dominant gene with partial penetrance. In atopic eczema the pattern of inheritance is not clearly defined and there is great variability in the degree to which associated conditions (asthma, hay fever, food allergies, and raised IgE levels) are present.

Skin conditions with autosomal *dominant* inheritance include neurofibromatosis, acute intermittent porphyria, tuberous sclerosis, and the less severe forms of ichthyosis and epidermolysis bullosa.

Autosomal *recessive* inheritance is responsible for the more severe forms of ichthyosis and epidermolysis bullosa as well as other rare diseases such as xeroderma pigmentosa.

X linked genes are responsible for rare disorders such as incontinentia pigmenti in which epidermal growth is abnormal. Blistering, warty, and pigmented lesions occur in whorls over the skin surface. These follow the lines of Blaschko, indicating the existence of a population of cells with a different X chromosome to the majority—an example of mosaicism. Central nervous system and skeletal abnormalities may be associated.

Recent advances in genetics, particularly gene mapping, are rapidly enlarging our understanding of the genetic basis of numerous diseases. This section indicates areas of relevance to dermatology that you may wish to pursue in larger texts.

FORMULARY

A great variety of preparations is available for treatment of skin conditions, and this list is limited to those in common use. There are numerous effective alternatives and it is inevitable that some medications have been omitted.

Topical treatment

General

The epidermis is capable of absorbing both greasy and aqueous preparations or a mixture of the two. The following should be used:
- Greasy ointments for dry scaling skin
- Watery creams for crusted weeping lesions
- Pastes where long action or occlusion is needed
- Gels for the face and scalp

Composition of bases

The consistency and properties of ointment and cream depend on the ratio of oil or grease to water (that is, whether they are oil in water or water in oil) and the emulsifying agents used—for example, emulsifying ointment contains soft white paraffin, emulsifying ointment and liquid paraffin.

The oils and greases range from mineral oil through soft paraffin to solid waxes. Some are naturally occurring, such as lanolin and beeswax. Creams or ointments may be used on their own as emollients or as vehicles for active ingredients.

Emollients—official preparations

Soft white paraffin—Greasy; protects skin and is long lasting.

Emulsifying ointment—Less greasy; mixes with water and can be used for washing.

Aqueous cream—Oil in water emulsion; useful as a vehicle, as an emollient, and for washing.

Liquid paraffin/white soft paraffin, equal parts—Spreads easily and is less greasy than white soft paraffin.

Hydrophilic ointment—Contains propylene glycol; mixes with water and spreads easily.

Lanolin (hydrous wool fat)—The natural emollient from sheep; mixes with water and greases, softens the epidermis, but can also cause allergic reactions.

Proprietary preparations

Proprietary preparations are numerous, varied, and more expensive than the standard preparations. They may also contain sensitisers—lanolin and preservatives (hydroxybenzoate, chlorocresol, sorbic acid)—and can cause allergies. Some examples are E45 cream (Crookes), Oilatum cream (Stiefel), and Lacticare (Stiefel), Unguentum Merck (Merck), Aquadrate (Norwich Eaton), and Diprobase (Scheing-Plough).

Both additives

Bath additives comprise dispersible oils such as Oilatum (Westwood, United States) Aveeno (Bioglan), Balneum (Merck), Alpha Keri, Westwood, United States), Emulsiderm (Dermal).

Tar preparations

Various vehicles are used, generally pastes as these remain on the skin longer and have a prolonged effect. In treatment centres the standard coal tar preparations can be used, but these are difficult to use at home. Coal tar paste contains a strong solution of coal tar of 7.5% in 25 g of zinc oxide, 25 g of starch, and 50 g of white soft paraffin.

In Edinburgh hospitals 0.5%–4% crude coal is used with 15% zinc oxide in yellow soft paraffin. It is easy to use and effective but has a strong, distinctive smell. A more pleasant mixture is 10% strong coal tar solution and 2% salicylic acid in Unguentum Merck. The salicylic acid helps to soften thick keratotic scales.

There are numerous proprietary preparations that are less messy and do not stain but are not so effective. They are useful for treating less severe psoriasis at home. Examples are: Alphosyl cream (Stafford-Miller), Pragmatar (Bioglan), Psoriderm (Dermal). Alphosyl HC (Stafford-Miller) and Carbo-Cort (Lagap) contain hydrocortisone as well.

Ichthammol is a useful soothing extract of shale tar. It can be made up as a 1% preparation in yellow soft paraffin with 15% zinc oxide.

Bath preparations

Bath preparations are useful for widespread psoriasis. Coal tar solution (20%) can be used or Polytar Emollient (Stiefel) or Psoriderm.

Tar shampoos are useful for treating psoriasis of the scalp. Polytar (Stiefel), T-Gel (Neutrogena), Capasal (Dermal), and Alphosyl (Stafford-Miller) are some examples.

Dithranol

Dithranol can be used in a paste containing salicylic acid, zinc oxide, starch, and soft white paraffin. It has to be applied carefully as it can cause severe irritation, avoiding contact with the surrounding skin.

For short contact treatment relatively clean preparations in a range of concentrations are available, such as Dithrocream (Dermal), Anthranol (Stiefel), and Psoradrate cream (Stafford-Miller).

Topical steroids

Topical steroids provide effective anti-inflammatory treatment but have the disadvantage of causing atrophy (due to decreased fibrin formation) and telangiectasis. They are readily absorbed by thin skin around the eyes and in flexures. On the face the halogenated steroids produce considerable telangiectasia so nothing stronger than hydrocortisone should be used (except in lupus erythematosus). They can cause hirsutism and folliculitis or acne. Infection of the skin may be concealed (Tinea incognita, for example) or made worse.

Side effects can be avoided by observing the following guidelines:
- Avoid long term use of strong steroids
- Potent or very potent steroids should be applied sparingly and often for a short time, then a less potent preparation less often as the condition improves
- Use only mildly potent steroids (that is, hydrocortisone) on the face
- Use preparations combined with antibiotics or antifungals for the flexures.

Topical steroids come in various strengths and a wide variety of bases—ointments, creams, oily creams, lotions, and gels—which can be used according to the type of lesion being treated.

Their pharmacological activity varies and they are classified according to their potency, the synthetic halogenated steroids being much stronger than hydrocortisone.
- Mildly potent —Hydrocortisone 0.5, 1, and 2.5%
- Moderately potent—Eumovate (Glaxo), Stiedex LP (Stiefel);
- Potent —Betnovate (Glaxo); Locoid (Brocades); and Synalar (ICI)
- Very potent —Dermovate (Glaxo).

In Britain a full list showing relative potencies appears in *MIMS*.

There are various combinations with antibiotics, antiseptic agents, and antifungals. Examples are: Terra-Cortril (Oxytetracycline, hydrocortisone) (Pfizer); Fucidin H (fucidic acid, hydrocortisone) (Leo); and Trimovate (Clobetasane butyrate, oxytetracycline, nystatin) (Glaxo).

Antiseptics and cleaning lotions

Simple antiseptics are very useful for cleaning infected, weeping lesions and leg ulcers.

Potassium permanganate can be used by dropping four or five crystals in a litre of water or in an 0.1% solution that is diluted to 0.01% for use as a soak. It will stain the skin temporarily and plastic containers permanently.

Silver nitrate 0.25% is a simple, safe antiseptic solution that, applied as a wet compress, is useful for cleaning ulcers.

Flamazine (Smith and Nephew) is silver sulphadiazine cream, used for leg ulcers, pressure sores, and burns.

Hydrogen peroxide (6%) helps remove slough but tends to be painful. Hioxyl (Quinoderm) is a proprietary cream for desloughing.

Iodine (2.5%) is an old fashioned effective preparation as a tincture in alcohol and Betadine (Napp) is a proprietary equivalent.

There are numerous other antiseptic, cleansing, and desloughing agents such as cetrimide, chlorhexidine, benzalkonium chloride, benzoic acid, and enzyme preparations such as Varidase (Lederle), a streptokinase and streptodornase preparation.

ACKNOWLEDGMENTS

Many colleagues have made useful comments on the ABC of Dermatology articles and, where appropriate, changes have accordingly been made to the text. In some cases, however, the points raised related to specialised or controversial aspects which could not be discussed at length within the limits of an ABC.

I am grateful to Dr Peter Ball, consultant in infectious diseases, Fife Health Board, for comments on infectious diseases, Dr M Jones, consultant in infectious diseases, City Hospital, Edinburgh, for comments on parvovirus infections, and Mr C V Ruckley, consultant surgeon, Royal Infirmary, Edinburgh, for comments on varicose ulcers.

Most of the illustrations are from the collection at the Victoria Hospital, Kirkcaldy, thanks to the expertise of Mr W McIntyre and his staff. Some are from the collection at the Royal Infirmary, Edinburgh, and a few were taken by the author.

The following colleagues kindly provided illustrations of specific conditions: Dr Peter Ball, rubella; Dr D H H Robertson, genital herpes; Mr C V Ruckley, varicose veins; Dr G B Colver, spider naevus; Dr M A Waugh and Dr M Jones, patients with AIDS; Professor R M Mackie, indirect immunofluorescence; and Dr P W M Copeman, common infections in black people.

P K B
Jan 1993

INDEX

Index

Index

Index